THE VIOLENT PERSON

Also by Raymond B. Flannery Jr., Ph.D., FAPM

Becoming Stress-Resistant through the Project SMART Program

Posttramatic Stress Disorder:
The Victim's Guide to Healing and Recovery (Second Edition)

Violence in the Workplace

Violence in America:
Coping with Drugs, Distressed Families,
Inadequate Schooling, and Acts of Hate

The Assaulted Staff Action Program (ASAP):
Coping with the Psychological Aftermath of Violence

Preventing Youth Violence:
A Guide for Parents, Teachers, and Counselors

THE VIOLENT PERSON

Professional Risk Management Strategies for Safety and Care

Raymond B. Flannery Jr., Ph.D., FAPM

2009

AMHF
AMERICAN
MENTAL
HEALTH
FOUNDATION
BOOKS

American Mental Health Foundation Inc
Post Office Box 3
Riverdale NY 10471-0003

www.americanmentalhealthfoundation.org

Library of Congress Cataloging-in-Publication Data

Flannery, Raymond B.
The violent person: professional risk management strategies for safety and care / Raymond B. Flannery Jr.
p. cm.
Includes bibliographical references and index.
ISBN-13: 978-1-59056-146-1 (hbk.)
ISBN-10: 1-59056-146-5 (hbk.)
ISBN-13: 978-1-59056-147-8 (pbk.)
ISBN-10: 1-59056-147-3 (pbk.)
1. Medical personnel—Violence against—Prevention.
2. Medical emergencies—Safety measures.
3. Violence. 4. Dangerously mentally ill. I. Title.
R727.2.F53 2009
616.02'5—dc22
2009019497

ISBN-13 978-1-935307-27-3 (hardcover)
ISBN-13 978-1-59056-147-8 (paperback)
E-Book ISBN-13 978-1-59056-148-5

For Those Who Serve
Others at Personal Risk to Themselves

Contents

Publisher's Foreword

As the present book is issued, The American Mental Health Foundation celebrates its 85th anniversary. Organized in 1924, AMHF is dedicated to the welfare of people suffering from emotional problems, with a particular concern for the emotional issues of those with special needs as well as the elderly. For many years, AMHF generally devoted its efforts to bettering quality of treatment and developing more effective methods, available even to low-income wage earners.

The major therapeutic advances and improved training methods are described in its existing publications: the series The Search for the Future. Two of these books are available on our Web site under the titles *The Challenge for Group Psychotherapy* (volume 1) and *The Challenge for Psychoanalysis and Psychotherapy: Solutions for the Future* (volume 2). (Portions of these books also are reprinted on the AMHF Web site in French and German, for a segment of the international community. These were prepared under the joint sponsorship of AMHF and the International Institute for Mental Health Research, Zurich and Geneva.) Volume 3, published by Prometheus Books in 2000, is entitled *Crucial Choices – Crucial Changes: The Resurrection of Psychotherapy.*

To date, all AMHF publications have appeared in at least three foreign languages.

Under the supervision and direction of Dr. William Van Ornum, AMHF Books is an exciting new venture. *The Violent Person* is by Dr. Raymond B. Flannery Jr., one of the foremost experts in the world on posttraumatic stress disorder (PTSD). We at AMHF are proud to make this book our first publication under our own imprint. The information in this clear-sighted work is not only for professionals. Anyone with a concern for and interest in the mechanisms of human violence and stress, in the workings of the human brain, would benefit from Dr. Flannery's jargon-free approach and decades of research and hands-on experience.

None of the board members of The American Mental Health Foundation receives remuneration. Nevertheless, the costs of promoting research, preparing translations, and disseminating the findings of AMHF are high. For this reason, all donations constitute a meaningful contribution to the public good. We thank you for helping us improve the lives of our citizens.

www.americanmentalhealthfoundation.org

Preface

A patient on the ward assaulted a staff member two hours ago. As you walk onto the floor now, are you safe? Your hospital beeper summons you to the emergency room to assess the condition of a drunken gang member. Do you survey the scene for safety as you enter the room? In your private practice office, you are assessing a patient with a known history of organic impairment and impulsivity. Have you thought to ensure your own safety? You are providing outreach to a troubled family with domestic violence. Are you at risk as you ring the doorbell? You are a youth outreach worker in the community. Are you in danger as you walk the streets? As you go about providing disaster relief services, do depressed and angry victim families present a risk of harm?

In recent years, our country has seen an unacceptable increase in human-inflicted violence. Health-care providers in all disciplines have not been immune from this violence. They have been victims of homicide, hostage-taking, robberies, physical and sexual assaults, verbal abuse, derogatory racial slurs, and psychological trauma, even as they were providing care to patients and clients. These attacks have been perpetrated in homes, on community streets, and at worksites, including private practice offices. Providing service for others in need is noble work but it has been becoming more inherently unsafe to do this work.

The violence inflicted by violent persons often occurs during behavioral emergencies when the potentially violent person is a patient or client in need of medical or psychiatric care. Behavioral emergencies are defined as critical incidents in which the patient's or client's medical or psychiatric crisis by its inherent nature also poses the risk of imminent, violent behavior toward the responding health care professional, the agitated victim, innocent family members, or bystanders. Common examples might include the drunken person severely cut by glass and in need of sutures or the person with paranoid schizophrenia who is hearing auditory hallucinations to kill others. These episodes of violence toward self or others may result from altered biological processes, impaired cognition and reasoning abilities and/or internal emotional distress. Environmental stressors often exacerbate these situations even further. The tasks in each behavioral emergency are twofold: (1) to provide the necessary medical or psychiatric care and (2) to do so in a way that reduces the risk of harm from the potentially violent person for all concerned.

Not every call for assistance is a behavioral emergency. However, some are, and we need to known how to provide needed services in ways that ensure the safety of everyone. Common potential behavioral emergencies include an array of medical illnesses as well as psychiatric emergencies such as psychosis, substance use, domestic violence, and youth violence. In addition, recent research has suggested that many of these behavioral emergencies themselves may also result in psychological trauma in the identified patients. Both the components of the original behavioral emergency and any resultant state of psychological trauma are both possible sources of violence that may confront the health care-provider as he or she provides assistance.

This book assumes that you have been well trained in the basic standards of practice that apply to the medical, psychological services or emergency services that you provide to patients or clients. In light of all of the fundamental information to be mastered, however, safety guidelines for managing behavioral emergencies may have received less attention during your training period. This book addresses this need for enhanced behavioral emergency safety training.

The first part of the book reviews the basic nature of behavioral emergencies and examines *general* strategies for assessing behavioral safety risks and for managing those risks, when they appear to be present. To further enrich our understanding of assessment and risk management strategies for behavioral emergencies, the first section of the book also contains a detailed review of what is known about why persons become violent.

With this as background information, the second section of the book provides an overview of four commonly encountered, potential behavioral emergencies: psychological trauma, domestic violence, psychiatric emergencies, and youth violence. These psychological behavioral emergencies may occur in their own right but may also be co-occurring in physical medicine emergencies as well. In each case, the psychological dimensions of the problem are reviewed and *specific* safety guidelines for that particular type of incident are presented. These specific guidelines supplement and expand on the general safety guidelines presented in the first section of the book.

Responding to behavioral emergencies is very stressful and can manifest its toll in our functioning at work and at home as well as in our physical and mental health. In the third section of the book, we examine important self-care issues to address this need. We will focus on several basic self-defense strategies that compliment the general and specific safety guidelines that have been outlined. Then, we will note some personal strategies for managing life and work stress, so that you may have good health and a sense of wellness. The sense of wellness is important to all of us so that we may continue to find our work enjoyable and satisfying. Finally, we shall practice implementing the various guidelines by examining the applications in several common clinical examples.

Since many professionals in all disciplines work in teams, a word of caution is in order. The safety of all of the members of the team or of an agency will be greatly enhanced, if all team members have read this book and discussed its strategies. In this way all team members will have some common understanding and agreement on how to address a particular behavioral emergency, so that team members will not be working at cross purposes during the emergency.

This book is based on the best-published research and standards of clinical practice and risk management approaches for professional health-care providers and emergency services personnel. It is written in practical, nontechnical language so that guidelines may be easily, safely, and quickly retained in memory. This book may also be of interest to the general reader with an interest in violence. It will help the general reader understand the various types of violence, the contexts in which they occur, and why persons become violent. However, the safety and self-care guidelines require considerable clinical study and experience and should not be fielded by anyone in the absence of such training. This book may be kept in the ward, the clinic, the office, or medical evacuation unit so that it is available for quick review. It may also serve as a classroom text for those in formal training.

My hope for you is that these pages will provide you with helpful tools to enhance your safety and the quality of service that you provide, even in those situations in which the patient's or client's disorganization and potential for violence will need to be assessed and monitored as part of the overall care being provided. Behavioral emergencies may occur but violence does not need to come with the turf.

An author's intellectual roots are many and found in diverse sources. This book is immediately indebted to the community of scholars in medicine, behavioral science, and emergency services care who work quietly and in small steps to understand human behavior in general and human violence in particular. I am equally indebted to my patients and students in the past thirty-five years for what they have taught me about human-perpetrated violence and its severe impact on human health.

My appreciation is also expressed to the following men and women who have more directly influenced the development of this book: Carl Bielack, R.N.; Jack Burke, M.D.; Joseph Coyle, M.D.; George Everly Jr.; Ph.D.: Thomas Grisso, Ph.D.; M. Annette Hanson, M.D.; Elaine Hill; Donald Howell; Norma Julin; Jeffrey Lating, Ph.D.; Barbara Leadholme, M.S., M.B.A.; Richard Levenson, Psy. D.; Jeffrey T. Mitchell, Ph.D.; Anthony Riccitelli; Marcia Scott, M.D.; John Terry, Ph.D.; James A. Woods, S.J., Ed.D.; Victor Welzant, Psy.D.; and Douglas Zedonis, M.D. Special thanks are also extended to my publisher, Evander Lomke, and to my wife, Georgina J. Flannery, M.S., reference librarian, research associate, teacher, and caring spouse. Without her this book would not be. I would also like to close by noting that it is an honor to be the first book published by the distinguished American Mental Health Foundation.

All of these men and women have provided thoughtful and wise suggestions. However, any errors remain my sole responsibility.

This book is dedicated to the professionals in all disciplines who quietly and in self-effacing ways serve others in need, even in those situations that place their own lives and safety at risk.

Raymond B. Flannery Jr., Ph.D., FAPM
Autumn 2008

Author's Note and Editorial Method

Human violence is a rapidly expanding area of scientific and medical inquiry. As with any aspect of health care, medications and interventions are continuously being improved. This book provides information on risk management strategies that have proven helpful with some violent patients in some situations. These strategies may not work in every instance and are not meant to be the answer in every situation. They are also not meant to replace what is currently working for you and your colleagues. Always follow your own judgment and whatever policies and trainings that your organization has provided. If you are working as a team, be sure that every team member is in agreement on how to approach the patient or client. As with the risk management strategies, the nonviolent self-defense releases outlined here are presented only as examples of possible options. They are not a substitute for formal training in these matters and the author is not responsible for your employing these risk management strategies and/or releases without such adequate training by skilled experts.

Note carefully the specific suggestions and warnings for the relaxation and aerobic exercises in the Appendixes. For the aerobic exercises, everyone is advised to begin with a medical exam to obtain medical clearance. Raise any questions that you may have with your physician and always follow his or her advice.

All chapter vignettes and clinical examples in the book are based on composites of several similar incidents, and all potentially identifying information has been further altered to protect the confidentiality of those involved.

A References and Select Reading list has been provided at the end for further reading as well as for all of the citations in the book. Citations in the text are listed by name(s) and year of publication and may similarly be found in the Readings list.

In this book, professionals, health-care providers, and/or caregivers refer to those who provide emergency medical and psychiatric care. These include physicians, surgeons, psychiatrists, psychologists, nurses, social workers, school psychologists, pastoral counselors, care managers, residential house staff, youth workers, the spectrum of emergency services providers, and others in similar work.

PART ONE

The Violent Person: Assessment/Risk Management

ONE

Assessment/Risk Management

Hope is necessary in every condition.

—Samuel Johnson

It felt as if one were in a furnace. Ninety-three degree heat, tropical humidity, sun-drenched pavement, no shade. Tanya stood alone on the concrete in this heat. Her own thirst was made worse by the fact that she had no medicine for her diabetes. She clutched beside her in a white sheet her most treasured possession.

She was on an overpass. Both ends of the overpass had been swept away by the winds and rains of Hurricane Katrina and now there was no way out. The tidal surges had left her on an island, a cement island that was surrounded by water contaminated by decaying bodies, raw sewerage, and poisonous chemicals.

Chaos was the only order in this municipal descent into hell. Fightings, shootings, lootings, burning buildings in a sea of water. Search and rescue, later search and recovery, helicopters at roof top levels.

She wondered if help would come in time or if she would die on this concrete slab. At least, they would be together. She wondered also how she would handle the bloating, the discoloration, and the gangrene. Thirty years and it had come to this. Perfect love did not always make it easy but with no funeral directors, no ministers, and no cemeteries, what was she to do?

With circumspection she opened the white sheet that held the only possession that she had left, her deceased husband, who had drowned pushing her to safety. She gently held his hand.

No. Death would not part them in this sea of chaos.

If you were the responding professional health care-provider and were confronted with the urban chaos and violent persons noted above, what would you do to assist? Where would you begin? What steps would you take to assure your own safety, as you provided care to others, given the shootings, lootings, and other forms of civil disobedience that surrounded you?

As noted in the preface, behavioral emergencies are defined as critical incidents in which the nature of the incident itself not only requires medical or psychiatric attention but at the same time also poses the risk of imminent, violent behavior toward the responding health care-provider, the agitated victim, innocent family members, or bystanders. These forms of behavioral dysregulation may arise from altered biological processes (e.g., substance use), impaired cognitive and reasoning ability (e.g., psychosis), and/or intense, negative emotions (e.g., domestic violence rage). Environmental stress, such as that of the hurricane and its aftermath in the present example, may further exacerbate already compromised functioning, as will any resultant psychological trauma.

Thus, when professionals arrive onsite, it is important that all of us be as thoroughly prepared as possible for potential violence and the steps needed to reduce its risk. This first section of the book speaks to this issue directly in terms of fundamental, general safety strategies. This first chapter examines the general nature of behavioral emergencies and reviews basic assessment/risk management strategies to prevent, mitigate, and/or contain violence, when we come upon it. The second chapter in this section provides an overview of the theories of human-perpetrated violence, so that we may better understand what motivates patients to become aggressive. Understanding the person's motivation provides us with additional tools to defuse critical incident tension.

We begin by examining the research findings that spell out clearly that we are at potential risk as we set about helping others in crisis.

The Nature of Behavioral Emergencies

The research on violence against health-care providers is largely reported for psychiatric patients and documents patient violence toward staff as a continuing, nationwide occupational hazard. There are two classes of patients that are more likely to be violent in both hospital and community settings. The first is the older male patient with a diagnosis of schizophrenia or other neurological abnormality and histories of violence toward others, and substance use disorder. The second grouping of patients are those persons with a diagnosis of personality disorder. These individuals are equally likely to be male or female, and have histories of violence toward others, personal victimization, and substance use disorders. Common precipitants to these assaults include acute psychotic disorganization, excess sensory overload, denial of services, and medication noncompliance. In hospitals, assaults occur most frequently between 7:00 A.M. and 9:00 A.M., when the ward is very active with meals, medications, showers, change-of-staff, and the like. In community residences, most assaults occur at 10:00 P.M., the most active hour in a community residence.

Additional research on violence and assaults on emergency services (EMS) personnel has documented this also to be a nationwide problem. Studies in Philadelphia, Chapel Hill, Nashville, Albuquerque, Sacramento, and Loma Linda have reported patient assaults in both home and non-home settings. The precipitants to these events have been medical emergencies, psychiatric disorganization, substance use disorders, gang conflicts, and the use of restraints. The Albuquerque study found that most assaults occurred between midnight and 6:00 A.M., where as in the Philadelphia study the high-risk period was logged between 6:00 P.M. and midnight.

It is important to note that this research has documented that health care and EMS personnel are not always at increased risk, even when responding to similar behavioral emergencies. There are times when the risk of assault by a patient may be greater or lesser. Recent research suggests that what appear to be random acts of violence may in fact not be random but follow specific temporal patterns, when looked at in the aggregate. Homicides seem to occur most frequently during the summer months. One-third of humanitarian workers die violently within the first ninety days of their service. Rapes appear to occur most commonly between 8:00 P.M. and 4:00 A.M. on Sunday evenings. Street assaults occur most often between 8:00 P.M. and 4:00 A.M. on any evening, whereas domestic violence occurs between 8:00 P.M. and 11:00 P.M. on weekends, twelve hours after the assailant has begun drinking heavily. On a similar note, most youth violence begins after 3:00 P.M., when school has let out for the day. School robberies occur most frequently when seventh-graders steal from other seventh-graders. This happens regularly in the United States, Canada, Japan, and Israel.

The research on violence against caregivers in the line of duty is clear, compelling, and concise. Each behavioral emergency carries within it the imminent risk for violence that we ignore at our own peril. Whether it is our first incident or our one-thousandth incident, we always want to assess for the warning signs of potential loss of control and, if noted, move quickly with appropriate risk management strategies to defuse the situation. (For those interested in reading this summarized research in greater detail, these studies with their full original references may be found in Flannery, White, Flannery, and Walker [2007].)

General Assessment/Risk Management Strategies

With these research findings as a backdrop, we now want to focus our attention on general assessment/risk management strategies to enhance our capacity to deal with potential patient violence. We will examine the medical conditions associated with violence, the importance of the patient's admitting chart for health-care providers and the case log for EMS, surveying the scene, recognizing old brain stem functioning in the patient or client, and evaluating any individual for the early warning signs of potential loss of control.

Medical Conditions and Violence

Tables 1 and 2 present the most common medical and psychiatric illnesses that are associated with potential patient violence. These listings are not meant to be exhaustive but do represent many of the most common situations in which behavioral emergencies may arise. In addition, there are some other rare medical issues that may also be associated with violence. These include severe vitamin deficiencies, toxins, sleep disorders, limbic encephalitis, and Wilson's disease (Tardiff, 1998).

Thus, the first intervention for safety is to consider the medical issue that you are being asked to respond to. Apart from anything else, first and foremost, ask yourself whether this person's medical condition is associated with possible violence.

The Patient's Admitting Chart/The Call Log

Most of us would probably not think of the patient's admitting chart or the EMS call log as safety tools. However, if they are properly constructed, they may well be an additional tool in the effort to reduce the risk for violence. These two sources of patient information before care is provided may help to identify potential behavioral emergencies and possible violence, may reveal timing patterns in potentially violent situations that at first appear to be random, and may assist in developing staffing levels for high risk periods.

To serve these purposes, the log or admitting chart needs to record relevant information on the identified patient, the responding agency staff, the environmental context, the time of the event, and other salient variables for a specific agency's mission. Health care, EMS, schools, and the like, may all benefit from a comprehensive approach to gathering initial information. This information may be especially helpful in dealing with potentially violent, frequent-service utilizers. The report form is most likely to be completed, if it can be done quickly. Check-off boxes on the sheet may be helpful toward this end and enhance staff compliance. Admitting records and logs can be updated and modified easily as better information is gleaned from the population served. When the paper form is completed, the

TABLE 1. Medical Illnesses Associated with Potential Violence

Akathesia	*Lupus*
Alzheimer's Disease	*Multi-Infarct Dementia*
Cushing's Disease	*Multiple Sclerosis*
Delirium	*Normal Pressure Hydrocephalous*
Glycemic Conditions	*Parkinson's Disease*
Head Trauma, Traumatic Brain Injury	*Pick's Disease*
Hepatic/Renal Disease	*Porphyria*
Hypovolemia	*Seizures*
Hypoxia Due to Cardiac/ Respiratory Illness	*Stroke*
Infections	*Thyroid Condition*
Intracranial Bleed	*Tumors*

agency will need to develop a computer program to log each incident, so that over time possible patterns of violence may emerge.

Let me share an example with you. In 1990, I created a crisis intervention program for health care staff that were assaulted by patients (Flannery, 1998). Known as the Assaulted Staff Action Program (ASAP), the program has logged assault incident data continuously for twenty years of service. It has taught us which patients are likely to assault, which staff are the likely victims, when and where these events will occur, and what is likely to precipitate each incident. It takes less than ten minutes to complete the ASAP log form and we have successfully modified it many times, as we have learned more about what information was most important to gather.

Figures 1 and 2 present both sides of the ASAP one-page report form and figures 3 and 4 present the computer data analysis form

TABLE 2. Psychiatric Illnesses Associated with Potential Violence

AIDS	*Oppositional Disorder*
Attention Deficit/ Hyperactivity Disorder	*Serious Mental Illness*
Conduct Disorder	*Shaken Baby Syndrome*
Dementia	*Somataform Disorder*
Domestic Violence	*Street Crime*
Intermittent Explosive Disorder	*Substance Use*
Mental Retardation	*Suicide*
Personality Disorder (Antisocial, Borderline, Narcissistic, Paranoid)	*Youth Violence*
Psychological Trauma and Posttraumatic Stress Disorder	*Violent Death*

onto which the report form data are entered. Each piece of information on the report form completed by the ASAP team member is entered into a corresponding block on the data entry sheet in figures 3 and 4. Each reported incident is entered on one line of data moving from left to right. Table 3 presents a summary of 2,152 incidents of patient assaults that the Massachusetts ASAP teams responded to over a fifteen-year period. This information has been useful in identifying high risk situations and staffing accordingly, and in providing risk information for new hires and for all employees during their annual re-certifications. With minimal staff time, the ASAP report form has yielded important information that has led to increased safety and reduced risk from harm. With a similar patient admitting form or call log, your agency can equally benefit from the information that it gathers.

FIGURE 1. ASAP: The Assaulted Staff Action Program

Date for 60/90 follow up:

Staff Victim: ______________ Date: __________ Job Block/Position: __________

Shift: __________ Time: __________ Unit: __________ Result of Restraint: __________

Description of Assault: ______________________________

Injuries: ___ ASAP Injury codes: 1 – Soft tissue (with/without swelling); 2 – Head or back; 3 – Bone/tendon/ligament; 4 – Open wound/scratches/bites; 5 – Spitting; 6 – Abdominal trauma; 7 – Psychological fright; 8 - No distress.

Severity: ___Severity rating (as determined by victim & ASAP member): 1 – None – No appreciable medical injury and/or psychological distress; 2 – Mild – Mild medical injury and/or psychological distress; 3 – Moderate – Moderate medical injury and/or moderate psychological distress; 4 – Serious – Serious medical injury and/or psychological distress; 5 – Intense – Intense medical injury and/or psychological distress.

Action Taken/Results: ______________________________

Staff Victim Response: ______________________________

ASAP Team Member(s) responding: __________ Signature: __________

__________ Signature: __________

Time & Date of Notification: __________ Time & date of First Contact: __________

Characteristics of Assaultive Patient

Age: _____ Sex: _____

Date of Adm: ______

Nbr of Adm: ______

History of:

___ substance abuse?

past ___ present ___ both ___

___ violence towards others?

___ past violent abuse in patient's own life?

___ substance abuse at the time of assault?

___ patient section

___ previous assault on unit? (Yes/No)

Primary Diagnosis:

1 - Schizophrenia

2 - Bipolar Illness (Manic/Depressive)

3 - Major Depressive Episode

4 - Personality Disorder Type: __________

5 - Substance Abuse only

6 - Organic Brain Dysfunction

7 - Other: __________

Specify: __________

Precipitants:

1 - Denial of Service

2 - Med. Noncompliance

3 - Excess sensory stim.

4 - Misdirected affection

5 - Negative staff attitude

6 - Court commit. ext'n

7 - Acute psychosis

8 - Other:

Specify: __________

FIGURE 2

Notes: ____

____

____

Mastery: (Staff victim is...)	1st	2nd	3rd
➪ Visibly shaken	☐	☐	☐
➪ Choosing to leave worksite	☐	☐	☐
➪ Medically injured and must leave worksite	☐	☐	☐
➪ Reporting feeling overwhelmed & out of control	☐	☐	☐
➪ Reporting feeling surprised but, otherwise, fine	☐	☐	☐
➪ Dismissing incident and seems in control	☐	☐	☐
➪ Dismissing incident, saying "it comes with the turf"	☐	☐	☐
➪ Appearing to need help, but refuses offer	☐	☐	☐
➪ Using denial totally	☐	☐	☐
➪ Other (specify)	☐	☐	☐

Meaning: (Staff victim is...)	1st	2nd	3rd
➪ Not attributing violence to psychosis	☐	☐	☐
➪ Not attributing violence to recent known event in patient's life (i.e. visit by family)	☐	☐	☐
➪ Not attributing violence to changes in hospital	☐	☐	☐
➪ Not attributing violence to the assault being part of the job	☐	☐	☐
➪ Unable to make meaningful sense of what has happened	☐	☐	☐
➪ Other:	☐	☐	☐

Attachments: (Staff victim is...)	1st	2nd	3rd
➪ Unable to turn to other staff	☐	☐	☐
➪ Unable to turn to unit managers	☐	☐	☐
➪ Unwilling to come to staff victim's support group	☐	☐	☐
➪ Unable to turn to family	☐	☐	☐
➪ Not able to identify an adequate or desired support network of any form	☐	☐	☐
➪ Other:	☐	☐	☐

Physical Symptoms: (Staff victim is...)	1st	2nd	3rd
➪ Hypervigilant	☐	☐	☐
➪ Experiencing exaggerated startle response	☐	☐	☐
➪ Having difficulty sleeping	☐	☐	☐
➪ Having difficulty with concentration	☐	☐	☐
➪ Experience mood irritability (especially anger and depression)	☐	☐	☐

Avoidant Symptoms: (Staff victim is...)	1st	2nd	3rd
➪ Avoiding specific thoughts, feelings, activities or situations	☐	☐	☐
➪ Diminished interest in significant activities	☐	☐	☐
➪ Restricted range of emotions (numbness)	☐	☐	☐

Intrusive symptoms: (Staff victim is...)	1st	2nd	3rd
➪ Describing recurring, distressing recollections (thoughts, memories, dreams, nightmares, flashbacks)	☐	☐	☐
➪ Describing physical or psychological distress at event that symbolizes the trauma	☐	☐	☐
➪ Describing grief or survivor guilt	☐	☐	☐

Three day follow-up. Date: __________ Staff victim response: ____________________

____

____

Ten day follow-up. Date: __________ Staff victim response: ____________________

____

____

FIGURE 3. Developing a Case Log

First Response	Avoidant Symptoms										
	Intrusive Symptoms										
	Physical Symptoms										
	Meaning										
	Attachments										
	Mastery										
VICTIM / DATE	Precipitant										
	Patient Section										
	Previous Assault on Unit (Y/N)										
	Ward CISD										
	Staff group										
	Restraint and Seclusion (Y/N)										
	Severity										
	Injuries III										
	Injuries II										
	Injuries I										
	Type of Assault										
	ASAP Team member										
	Refused ASAP contact? (Y/N)										
	Prior ASAP contact? (Y/N)										
	Date of Assault - Year										
	Date of Assault - Day										
	Date of Assault - Month										
	Time of Day (use 24 hour time, i.e. 1630 for 4:30 p.m.)										
	Shift										
	Unit										
	Sex of Staff Victim										
	Job Block										
	Staff Victim Number										
	Hospital Group Number										

ASAP PROGRAM NUMBERS

1 - Taunton
2 - Medfield
3 - Westborough
4 - Worcester
5 - Tewksbury
6 - Metro Boston Shelters
7 - Quincy MHC
8 - Center for MH
9 - Cambridge-Somerville
10 - Bay Cove MHC
11 - Pocasset MHC
12 - Carney Hospital
13 - MBMHSU of LSH

JOB BLOCK:

1 - MHW
2 - RN
3 - LPN
4 - Pyschologist
5 - REC Therapist
6 - Social Worker
7 - Psychiatrist
8 - OT Therapist
9 - Lab Tech
10 - MD
11 - RC
12 - House Manager
13 - Case Manager
14 - Clinician
15 - Allied Mental Health
16 - Support Staff
(ie: housekeeping, clerical)
17 - Student
18 - OTHER

SHIFT:

1 - 7A-3P
2 - 3P-11P
3 - 11P-7A

DAY OF WEEK:

1 - Sunday
2 - Monday
3 - Tuesday
4 - Wednesday
5 - Thursday
6 - Friday
7 - Saturday

RESTRAINT:

0 - No
1 - Yes
2 - Unknown

GENDER CODES:

1 - Female
2- Male

PRIMARY DIAGNOSIS OF PATIENT:

1 - Schizophrenia
2 - Bipolar Disorder
3 - Major Depressive Episode
4 - Personality Disorder
5 - Substance Abuse Order
6 - Organic Brain Dysfunction
7 - Other - Specify: ______________

____

____

PT HISTORY OF VIOLENCE AS A VICTIM:

0 - No
1 - Yes
2 - Unknown

YES/NO QUESTIONS:

0 - No
1 - Yes
2 - Unknown

DESCRIPTION OF ASSAULT:

1 - Physical Assault
2 - Sexual Assault
3 - Non-verbal Threats
4 - Verbal Threats/Racial slurs
5 - Other: ____________________

____

____

____

ASAP INJURY CODE:

1 - Soft tissue injury
(with/without swelling)
2 - Head or back injury
3 - Bone/tendon/ligament injury
4 - Open wound/scratches/bites
5 - Spitting
6 - Abdominal trauma
7 - Psychological fright
8 - No distress

SEVERITY:

1 - None
2 - Mild
3 - Moderate
4 - Serious
5 - Intense

FIGURE 4. Developing an Admitting or Case Log

ASSAULTIVE PATIENT	Assaultive Patient:										
	History of Violence as Victim										
	History of Violence towards Others										
	Substance Abuse (past history)										
	Substance Abuse (@ time of assault)										
	Primary Diagnosis										
	Age										
	Sex										
Third Encounter	Avoidant Symptoms										
	Intrusive Symptoms										
	Physical Symptoms										
	Meaning										
	Attachments										
	Mastery										
Second Encounter	Avoidant Symptoms										
	Intrusive Symptoms										
	Physical Symptoms										
	Meaning										
	Attachments										
	Mastery										

PATIENT SECTION:

1 - Sect. 7 & 8
2 - Sect. 10
3 - Sect. 11
4 - Sect. 12
5 - Sect. 13
6 - Sect. 15A
7 - Sect. 15B
8 - Sect. 15E
9 - Sect. 16A
10 - Sect. 16B
11 - Sect. 18A
12 - Sect. 18B
13 - None
14 - Other ______________________

PRECIPITANTS:

1 - Denial of Services
2 - Med. noncompliance
3 - Excess Sensory Stim.
4 - Misdirected affectation
5 - Negative staff attitude
6 - Court commit. extension
7 - Acute psychosis
8 - Other (specify) ______________

TABLE 3. Developing an Admitting or Case Log

Assaultive Psychiatric Patients: Fifteen-year Findings of the Assaulted Staff Action Program (ASAP)

This statistical summary is based on 2,152 MA Department of Mental Health cases over the fifteen-year period from 1990–2005:

Inpatient Assaults: Staff most at risk continue to be new, less experienced, less formally trained mental health workers and nurses during restraint and seclusion procedures. The assaultive patient is most likely to be of the same gender; to have a primary diagnosis of schizophrenia or personality disorder; to have past histories of violence toward others, personal victimization, and substance use disorder. The most likely precipitants are acute psychosis, denial of services, and/or excess sensory stimulation. Such assaults are most likely to occur in the middle ten days of the month on the first shift from 7:00-9:00 A.M.

Community Assaults: Staff most at risk include new, less experienced mental health workers and residential house staff and nurses during restraint procedures. The assaultive patient is most likely to be of the same gender; to have a primary diagnosis of schizophrenia or personality disorder; to have past histories of violence toward others, personal victimization, and substance use disorder. The most likely precipitants are acute psychosis, denial of services, and/or excess sensory stimulation. Such assaults are likely to occur in the first ten days of the month. In community mental health centers these assaults are most likely to occur on the first shift from 7:00-9:00 A.M. In community residences, the most likely time of assault is on the second shift between 10:00-11:00 P.M.

Surveying the Scene

In terms of safety, when you are summoned to a site to provide care, it is critical that you are *scene-oriented* first and then *patient-oriented.* Each of us needs to be sure that we have evaluated the scene for potential or actual risks for violence before we turn our attention to patient needs. Police officers are routinely trained in scene surveillance. Some, but not all, EMS are trained in scene surveillance. However, health care professionals are rarely trained in scene surveillance. Below is a short outline of the main points to be considered in approaching a home and a vehicle on the street where help has been requested. (Further detailed training may be obtained in conjunction with local policing agencies and in excellent books on the subject by D. Krebs [2003] and Mitchell and Resnick [1981]. Books by P. M. Kleepsies [1998] and K. Tardiff [1996)] contain some surveillance implications for health care professionals.)

Preliminary Considerations. Before you are called upon to provide assistance, you want to prepare as much in advance as you can. For health care professionals, you want to know some system of nonviolent self-defense, have reviewed the alternatives to restraint and seclusion, and have some system for summoning aid quickly, should it prove necessary. For EMS, this includes not looking like police officers (no badges, uniforms in the colors of local police), having a walkie-talkie with a panic button that has been frequency tested, wearing reflective gear, and knowing your cop car. Neither group should wear neckties, jewelry, or have on their person any garment or object that could be used as a weapon against them. In both groups, if you are entering a high crime area, go with the police or arrange some way to summon them quickly.

Entering a Building. If you have been asked to provide assistance with a medical or psychiatric illness in a home, you need to survey the street first, then the outside of the home, and then the inside of the home. Remember: scene before patient. If you are harmed, the patient will not receive your attention.

If it is geographically possible, begin on the street behind the address that you have been called to and see if it is safe in the back of that building. (EMS should shut down lights and sirens several blocks away to retain the element of surprise.) Is anyone in the back? Is anyone hiding? Can you explain to yourself why any and all particular persons might be there? Next, drive to the street from where the call has come. As you approach the identified street address to provide assistance, drive slowly past the building, so that you can see all remaining three sides. Can you explain to yourself why various people may be there? Bystanders? Neighbors? Troublemakers? Gang members? Continue to survey the street. Look up at balconies, behind trees and mailboxes, and similar places and objects to be sure that it is safe. Park beyond the house in question and leave yourself a street exit.

Next, approach the house and its doors from the sides of the building. Do not walk up the front entrance way. Listen for sounds of possible violence inside. Open the door from the side and never shut the door. Step in quickly and move to the sides of the door so that you are not in harm's way. Keep your back to the wall and then scan the interior for weapons, potential weapons, and possible assailants. (If you approach a house at night with a flashlight, hold the light to your side so that you are not silhouetted.) If you came up by elevator, lock the elevator on the floor you are on and look for other exits out of the building that you are in. Ask that potential weapons be removed. Observe others in the room for potential signs of loss of behavioral control (see below); then, turn your attention to the patient.

If there is a team of two, a "care and cover" approach is best. One member provides needed patient care and the other continuously observes the room and its occupants. No one is left alone or leaves the room alone. In medical situations, search for weapons on the patient as part of a physical exam. If at any step in this process caregivers feel unsafe and sense danger, they should summon police assistance.

Vehicle in Street. Park several feet behind the vehicle at a ten-degree angle to the curb so that your engine block can serve as a shield. On night calls, flash your high beams into the vehicle's rear and side view mirrors so that the occupant(s) cannot see you coming. Approach the vehicle fifteen to twenty feet away from it on its passenger side. Note trees, utility poles, mailboxes, hydrants and similar objects that you can use for cover, if necessary, Move to the trunk and be sure the trunk is locked. Then, move to the right rear fender and survey any occupants and contents in the rear seat. If that appears safe, move to the car's door support column and do a similar search of the front seat area. Assess for any attempt by the driver or other front seat occupant to reach under the dashboard for a weapon and be prepared to take cover. If there seems to be no immediate potential for harm, use the "care and cover" approach in treating the patient. Both care and cover are important. In one recent example, a paramedic was providing care to a car accident victim in the middle of the street. He was suddenly pummeled on his head with high-heeled shoes by an angry female driver who was behind the medivac unit and who was outraged that the unit was blocking the street.

In any situation where you find the patient face down with his or her hands underneath the person's body, immediately check the patient's hands for possible weapons used against the self, others, or both.

As you can see from this brief discussion, scene surveillance is an important part of addressing possible behavioral emergencies. I recommend that each reader study the books noted above and speak with local police to review these and more detailed procedures. There is no substitute for scene safety in the face of potentially violent persons.

The Old Brain Stem

Figure 5 presents a rough outline in side-view of some of the major structures in the brain and we will refer to these now and later in the book. The cortex is our thinking brain. Here we receive messages from our senses, review memory to see if we have encountered this situation before, make a decision about what to do, and then implement our coping strategies. The prefrontal cortex is in the area of our forehead and it is where the brain makes its decisions about what to do. The limbic system is that part of the brain that adds feeling tone to experience. If I am looking at a dog and my past experiences with dogs have been pleasant ones, I will have

FIGURE 5. The Basic Structure of the Brain

STRESS ⟶ THE OLD BRAIN STEM

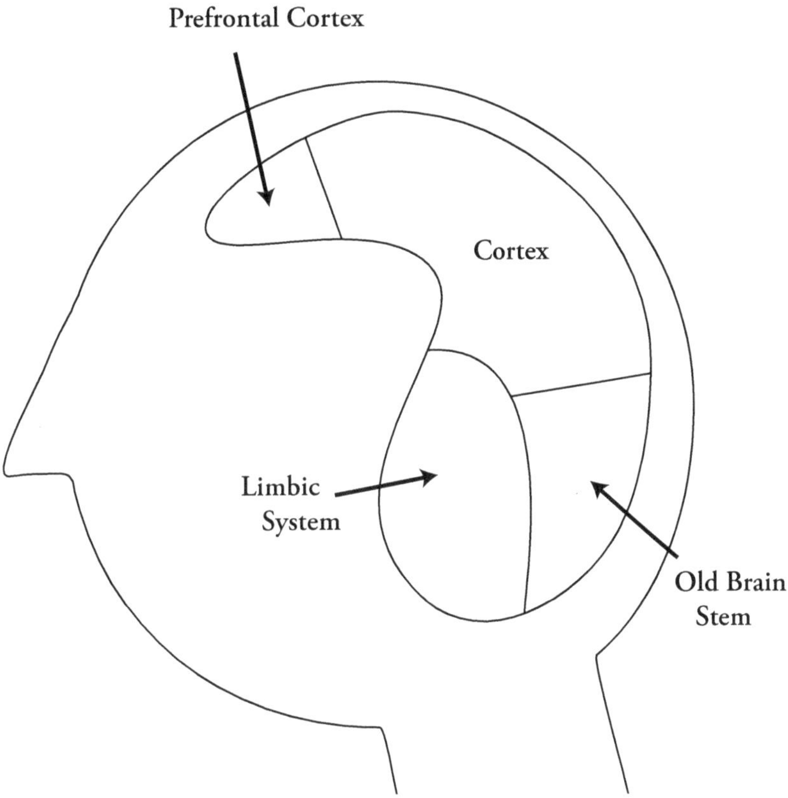

feelings of calmness and happiness in my limbic area. However, if my experiences with dogs have been frightening, then I will experience fear in my limbic area. Lastly, the old brain stem is the seat of all of our vital functions that keep us alive, such as breathing, sleeping, feeling hungry. Much of our instinctual behavior is rooted in the old brain stem.

In some situations, when a person is under severe stress, immediate functioning moves from the cortex to the old brain stem, so that individuals under stress may react quickly, more from force of habit, rather than from detailed cognitive reasoning. Behavioral emergencies may result in the patient or client functioning at an old brain stem level. To assess the patient's or client's needs and to enhance quality of our care, we want to return the patient to higher cortex functioning. This is done by simple messages that are paced slowly over the first few minutes. This reduces the patient's level of stress and provides a breathing space, so that the patient may reorient him- or herself and begin to think more fully, as the prefrontal cortex reasserts its prominence. Some simple statement relevant to the situation, such as "Let's take a moment" followed by a long pause and then repeated with another long pause two more times, gives the patient a chance to readjust. Restoring higher cognitive functioning enhances safety and assists in providing care. This process may be helpful in beginning to defuse some behavioral emergencies.

Warning Signs of Loss of Control

Table 4 outlines some of the early warning signs of impending loss of control and should be remembered by all of us who respond to behavioral emergencies. These warning signs are grouped into three categories: medical disorders, appearance, and behaviors.

Medical disorders that we know to be associated with possible violence (see figures 1 and 2) should always be considered as potential sources of violence in any given patient or client that we are working with, even if the person appears calm as we begin. The appearance of the patient is the second area to explore for possible impending loss of control. Is the patient disorganized or tense? Does he or she have glazed eyes due to possible drug use? Is the individual wearing sunglasses to hide paranoid fears? Are long sleeves covering drug tracks on an arm? Each of these factors may indicate a person in tenuous control with possible old brain stem functioning.

Lastly, the behavioral factors, again, are measures of impending loss of possible control. Severe agitation with pacing or wring-

TABLE 4. Warning Signs of Loss of Control

1. *Medical Disorders Associated with Aggressive Outbursts*

2. *Appearance*
   - Disorganized in Physical Dress or Appearance
   - Tense Facial Expressions
   - Glazed Eyes
   - Inappropriate Use of Dark Glasses
   - Long Sleeves in Hot Weather

3. *Behavior*
   - Behavioral Signs of Severe Agitation
   - Verbally Hostile and Argumentative
   - Suggestions of Substance Use
   - Verbal Threats to Specific Persons
   - Threat of Weapons

ing of hands, verbally hostile interactions, possible substance use further disinhibiting the control centers in the brain, and specific threats to others are all signs of persons in very tenuous control. A good rule of thumb is this: the more the warning signs, the greater the likelihood of loss of control. Interventions to move the person from old brain stem to higher cortex functioning may help to calm the situation.

Not all emergencies lend themselves to detailed discussions with the patient. However, health-care providers, if they have time in any given instance, may want to consider five screening questions that Borum, Swartz, and Swanson (1996) have found helpful in assessing and managing violence risk. Ask if the patient has trouble controlling his or her temper; does the person hit people or damage property when he or she is angry; what is the most violent thing the person has done; what is the closest the person has come to being violent; does the person fear physically harming someone? The person's answers to these questions can help you gauge the immediacy of risks.

This completes the overview of general strategies for the assessment and risk management of behavioral emergencies that may present with the potential for violence by the patient, the patient's family, or friends. We want to routinely remember: to consider the medical or psychiatric illness that we have been asked to report to; to gather any relevant information from the patient admitting log or call log; to survey the scene, as we arrive onsite; to consider that old brain stem functioning may be prominent; and to monitor the patient or client for any of the early warning signs of potential loss of control.

If we return to our chapter example of the hurricane in light of these safety guidelines, what might we learn about potential risks of violence toward caregivers who respond with assistance? The identified victim has two medical conditions associated with potential violence, diabetes and the profound grief at the violent death of her husband. We probably would not have specific log information on this poor woman but we would have recorded in the log specific information about the types and frequencies of the violence that surround her in the city and possibly some information on the characteristics of the assailants of the street crimes. With this information we could make a more thorough survey of the scene, evaluate the possible prominence of old brain stem functioning in our patient, and check for the presence of any of the common warning signs of potential loss of control. These general basic guidelines would greatly enhance our capacity to complete a thorough assessment and to establish risk management strategies for any potential patient violence. Safety is no accident.

The epigraph at the beginning of the chapter spoke about the importance of hope in all situations and behavioral emergencies are no exception. We would need to provide to this overwhelmed patient some sense of hope that things can improve, that a decent burial for her husband can be had, and that the shattered pieces of her life can be stitched together, so that she may go on. It has been the experience of many professionals that the violence potential in many behavioral emergencies can be defused by moving the patient from old brain stem to cortex prominence and offering some measure of hope for the future.

Each chapter closes with a summary table of the main safety guidelines so that they may be easily remembered in times of crisis. Table 5 presents the principal general safety guidelines of the present chapter. We will add specific safety guidelines for differing behavioral emergencies, as we proceed through the book.

We turn our inquiry now to why persons in behavioral emergencies may become violent. An understanding of their motivations will lead to differing strategies to prevent or manage the violence. We turn now to the heart of darkness. How are we to understand why some human beings murder, maim, torture, and otherwise inflect pain on their fellow human beings?

TABLE 5. Safety Guidelines
Think Medical or Psychiatric Illness
Think Call Log
Think Scene Surveillance
Think Old Brain Stem
Think Early Warning Signs

TWO

Understanding Human Violence

Night and silence! Who is here?

—William Shakespeare

The door to the jail cell slammed shut. He was charged with vagrancy, disorderly conduct, and two charges of assault and battery on a police officer. So be it, he thought to himself. Life was not fair, the world was a jungle, and, as his voices had correctly predicted, no one could be trusted—not even the police.

Richard had grown up in a housing project on the other side of town. Both of his parents drank heavily and physically abused each other and himself. He tried to separate them during their fights, but he was small in stature and easily flung out of the way into nearby walls. He learned early on that the world was malevolent and that he should keep his head down and his guard up.

The voices had begun four years ago, when he was sixteen. These voices were his regular companions and their directives to harm himself or others were harsh and uncompromising. They particularly cajoled him to attack others first before those others came after him. He was frightened by the voices and had begun to use alcohol to calm his nerves.

Today's dark journey had played itself out at high noon. This morning his voices had been especially intense. He had used some alcohol to self-medicate, but with no measurable relief. He had gone to the park in search of solitude. However, his ill-kempt appearance and his constant pacing frightened nearby children and the police were called. The police surrounded him just as the voices had predicted that they would. This was the jungle made real.

The police told him to stand still. He was unable to stop from pacing. The police asked his name. He remained mute. One of the officers remembered the police academy instructor saying that, when communication fails, violence follows, but what do you do when the suspect will not speak? In the end, four officers rushed him. He lowered his head and fought as hard as he could. One officer sustained a broken wrist; a second, a scraped face.

Thus, the police had placed him in a cell and slammed shut the door. He wondered if they understood that in the jail cell of his schizophrenic illness the terror and loneliness were worse than anything the state had to impose.

When communication fails, violence follows.

Even though there is a good deal of violence in the world, when it erupts close to home in one's neighborhood by neighbors that everyone considered to be normal, people become frightened and confused. Violence teaches each of us how tenuous our links are to Mother Earth and murders, rapes, assaults, and the like remind us how vulnerable each of us truly is.

This chapter focuses on the evil of human-perpetrated violence on others and examines the various theories to explain such behavior. The initial response of many nonvictims is to assume that the violent person was out of his or her mind, as is the case in our chapter vignette. Yet, only a small percentage of human violence can be attributed to mental illness. This is a cold reality with which it is difficult to come to terms. In most instances, the violent acts were committed by violent persons who were not mentally ill and who were aware of what they were doing. Some behaved impulsively (behavior without thought) and, even worse, some behaved with premeditated, calculated hatred. In the latter case, the assailants clearly knew what they were about.

Why do people commit these heinous acts, including harming helpless children? What motivates or drives them to behave this way? The answer is complicated and not yet fully understood in medicine and science. However, behavioral science has developed and researched several theories that explain what may be at work in any given person's violent behavior. Often, more than one factor is at work in the same violent person.

Understanding what motivates a particular assailant is helpful information for those of us who respond to behavioral emergencies. Knowing, for example, that a person is intoxicated, seeking initiation into a local street gang, or suffering from infarct dementia provides us with information on how to differentially approach a particular patient or client to begin to defuse the risk for potential violence, so that safety for everyone is maintained.

There are four groupings of theories of violence: cultural, biological, sociological, and psychological and each is reviewed in due course. However, we will begin with the three basic principles of good physical and mental health because in each act of violence one or more of these domains is disrupted in the assailant. Moreover, each of these three domains also furnishes health-care providers with some basic intervention strategies to employ in defusing the potential for violence that is associated with their disruptions in behavioral emergencies.

The Domains of Good Health

Caring attachments to others, reasonable mastery in our lives, and a meaningful purpose in life are the three domains of human functioning that lead to good physical and mental health. Adequate functioning results in less anxiety and depression, less illness, and a sense of well-being. The absence of adequate functioning in these domains leads to the loss of a sense of well-being, increased illness, and a shortened lifespan. Anger and violence frequently accompany domain disruptions.

Caring Attachments to Others

Caring attachments are the meaningful bonds or links that we have with other humans. Humans are social animals and being close to others makes us feel good. The absence of others in our lives leads to a loneliness that can be very painful.

World War II in part provided the impetus to study the nature of human attachments. The war had disrupted many families through death, abandonment, and relocation. As families were torn apart, many children became orphaned and society did its best to understand how best to help these children. René Spitz (Lynch, 1977) was among the first to call attention to the importance of human contact and demonstrated how literally deadly could be its absence. In 1945-46, he studied ninety-one infants in orphanages in Canada and the United States. All of them were well cared for by staff but thirty-four died during the last three months of their first year of life. They wasted away in spite of good care and no obvious medical disease. Spitz wondered if the absence of the biological parent(s) in some way contributed to their early death.

During these same years, a British physician, J. Bowlby (1982), was also studying the importance of the mother for the growth of the child. It was obvious that a child was dependent on his or her parents for survival and for learning over time how to survive on its own. Bowlby felt that a child was born with a need to interact socially as a way of meeting these survival goals and Dr. Bowlby set about clarifying the nature of this process. Bowlby observed a child was content in the presence of its mother but, if the mother left the child, the child would scream in protest until its scream brought about the return of the mother and with her return the implications for safety. Bowlby called this mother/child bond an *attachment* and termed the child's distressed screaming in her absence a form of *separation anxiety*. He also noted that, in those cases where the mother did not return, the child would become despondent and depressed. The child remained detached from others, as if not wanting to be abandoned again. When the attachment was secure and consistent, the child's growth and development were normal and adaptive. In those cases where the attachment was insecure or absent, the child's growth was not normal and a variety of problems emerged over time.

Subsequent research has studied the nature of adult attachments. Attachments to family, friends and colleagues bring us companionship, emotional support in good times and bad, information about solving life-stressful problems, and instrumental favors in the forms of money or political influence on our behalf (see review in Flannery, 2004a). Other types of attachment, however, may prove to be harmful. These include those marked by physical or sexual abuse, emotional over involvement in others, emotional demanding-ness, interpersonal skill deficiency, and the like.

One additional important component of caring attachments is mastering the skills of empathy. Empathy refers to our ability to understand the feeling states of others. This process is usually begun in childhood when parents teach their offspring how other children and adults feel. For example, a mother might say to her child; do you remember when grandma died and you felt sad? Well, Jimmy's grandmother has died and he may feel sadness as you did, when your grandma died. This ability to walk in another person's shoes, to understand how they may be feeling forms the basis of empathy and is learned gradually over time. It is a complex skill.

It is also important in understanding some forms of violent behavior. Empathy forms the psychological basis for moral values to take root. Without empathy, it is rare for individuals to have true moral development. In some cases, the violent person harms another because the violent person has limited capacity to appreciate the suffering that he or she is inflicting on the victim.

In addition to the psychological components of caring attachments, physiologist, James Lynch (1977; 2000), was studying the physiological components of caring attachments at the same time as the psychological studies were being conducted. He found that a person's cardiovascular system (blood pressure and pulse), the person's immune system to fight upper-respiratory infections, and a person's endorphins endogenous opioid system (chemicals in the brain that make us feel good) were all strengthened in the presence of caring attachments. The reverse was true in socially isolated people. Indeed, he found that the absence of caring attachments resulted in premature death. Clearly, caring attachments are an important domain in good health.

Reasonable Mastery

Reasonable mastery refers to one's ability to shape the environment to meet one's needs. We learn work skills to earn money to eat, we learn social skills to make attachments, and so forth. These types of efforts enable us to pursue our goals in life and to enhance our quality of life, once we have met our basic goals.

Good problem-solvers have a basic set of cognitive strategies that they utilize to solve the issues and problems in life that confront them. First, they correctly identify the problem to be solved. If they are angry at something at work, they do not take that anger out on their family. Second, they gather information about how to solve the problem. They draw on past experience, reading, advice from friends, and the like. Third, they think out carefully specific solutions for the specific problem. They have more than one solution because they know that the world is complex and that their first solution may not work. Fourth, they implement the proposed solution, and, fifth, they evaluate it to see if it actually solved the problem.

Adaptive problem-solvers know something else. They know that they have the mental capabilities and physical strength to solve many problems in life but they also realize that total mastery of everything in life is unreasonable. Some problems they know they do not have the skills to solve. In other cases, they have tried their best but the problem remains unsolved. At some point, they know enough to stop trying and they put their energies to better use.

Poor problem-solving may result for many reasons, including medical or psychiatric illness, disability, inadequate parenting, poor schooling, or being emotionally overwhelmed and unable to think clearly.

Meaningful Purpose in Life

All of us need some reason to get up in the morning and invest our energies in the world around us. This purpose provides the motivation for us to move forward, especially during life's difficult moments. Many years ago, sociologist Aaron Antonovsky (1979) was the first to establish the importance of a sense of a coherent meaningful purpose in life. One's meaningful purpose needs to provide a sense of the world's manageability, to make the world comprehensible, and to provide a belief that the world is worthy of our investing energy in it. The components of the sense of coherence help us keep life in perspective and buffer the stress of life.

Humans are biological in part, yet have a conscious awareness of their own physical being. We know that our physical self will die at some point, so our conscious self tries to find a way to live on in the minds of others after our deaths. Thus, many successful meanings in life revolve around concern for others. These might include one's children, one's life-work, a community social cause, an artistic creation. This concern for others, in our meaningful purpose in life, is more robust than some of society's other proffered goals, such as money, power, fame, and fortune. These other worldly proffered goals all end in death and do not necessarily leave a legacy that is remembered by others. A meaningful purpose in life that is primarily centered on the self may result in an unnecessarily enhanced sense of self. This exaggerated sense of personal control will some day encounter a problem it cannot solve and at that point its sense of purpose may fail and serious depression may ensue.

Caring attachments, reasonable mastery, and a meaningful sense of purpose in life are the three domains of good health that foster normal moral childhood development and adaptive adult functioning. In the theories of violence to which we now turn, the domains are disrupted or absent and normal moral growth has not developed.

Theories of Human Violence

The theories of violence are many and varied and Table 1 presents a schematic overview of the most common explanations. No one single theory of violence can explain all of the various forms of violence and often there is more than one type of violence present in any given incident, as we have noted earlier. Understanding these various forms of violence may provide health care profession-

TABLE 1. Theories of Human Violence

Cultural:	Anomie
Biological:	Genetics Cortex/Limbic System Medical Illnesses
Sociological:	Poverty Inadequate Schooling Discrimination Domestic Violence Substance Use Easily Available Weapons The Media

Psychological:	Mastery
	   Personal Self-care Skills
	   Interpersonal Skills
	   Academic Skills
	Motivation

als with an awareness of what to expect and how to approach any given behavioral emergency. We begin with the cultural theories of violence because the presence of cultural roots of violence exacerbate the other three forms of violence. The interested reader will find these theories of violence discussed in much greater detail in Borak (2006), Defelm (2006), and Flannery (2000).

Cultural Theory

Culture may be defined as the customary beliefs, social forms, and material traits of a people. Although there have been many cultural theories of violence, the theory of Émile Durkheim (1858-1917) has gained the most prominence and many adherents.

Durkheim believed that culture exerted its influence through society's five basic social institutions: government, business, family, school, and religion. He saw these five institutions as the transmitters or educators of a culture's values and social norms. These institutions showed citizens what was expected, what was valued, how to be a productive member of society, and how to interact in socially approved ways with others. The adults then knew in turn the rules by which to raise their children. The end result of this process was an integrated social community in which people had caring attachments, reasonable mastery, and a meaningful sense of purpose. This adaptive regulation of social behavior led to a sense of cohesion in the community and a sense of belonging in the individual.

Durkheim's theory also predicted that, when a society underwent a major social upheaval, society's five basic social institutions would themselves undergo this upheaval, and the commonly agreed-upon set of rules to regulate social behavior among citizens would be in disarray. The sense of social cohesion and belonging would be lost. Durkheim referred to this state of loss as *anomie.* Durkheim supported his theory by reviewing all of the countries that had been through major social upheavals throughout history. He noted that after each upheaval the cohesion and sense of belonging were repeatedly replaced by increases in mental illness, substance use, suicides, and human-perpetrated violence toward others.

Many social scientists (e.g., Drucker, 1994) believe that we are in just such a major social upheaval in our own age. From 1850 until about 1970, our culture was referred to as the Industrial State. The Industrial State was characterized by the harnessing of energy to run machinery. At first, it was water to run spinning looms but subsequent advances in science and technology resulted in other forms of energy being coupled to machinery. Over time, coal, oil electricity, and atomic energy were harnessed to run everything from small appliances to motor vehicles and airplanes. The Industrial State became a society that produced goods and services based on ever expanding technological advances. Businesses expanded from small private ownership to multinational corporations and the general health and welfare of the people improved greatly during these years. These years were governed by a value system commonly known as the Protestant Work Ethic. It stressed concern for the welfare of others, especially the young and the elderly; hard work; honesty; self-control; self-denial to improve the lot of one's children; and sexual exclusivity in marriage. Although poverty and various types of discrimination remained, over time an increasing majority of citizens came to have caring attachments, reasonable mastery, and a sense of meaningful purpose that was rooted in concern for others.

The 1970s marked what Durkheim would see as a major social upheaval. Society moved from providing goods and services to creating knowledge after the advent of computers. Whereas an employee in the Industrial State might have physically made motor vehicles, in this new age, known as the *postindustrial state,* that same employee provided services and information by means of the computer. For example, an employee might enter insurance claims on a computer. The postindustrial state has seen the rise of three groupings of citizens: the knowledge workers who use the computers to make advances in understanding; the service workers who provide the resources and support to keep the knowledge workers efficient; and the permanent underclass who are unschooled and unskilled and, therefore, unable to join one of the first two groups. Moreover, a new value system has emerged to replace the Protestant Work Ethic. Postindustrial values emphasize the self first, material goods, and instant gratification.

As Durkheim foresaw, the five major societal institutions have themselves been caught up in this transition. The common agreement on acceptable social behavior has been lost with a resultant decline in the sense of community cohesion and belongingness. Mental illness, substance use, suicide, and violence toward others have all increased in our age and many of today's citizens do not have caring attachments, reasonable mastery, or a meaningful sense of purpose. It is likely that this transition to the postindustrial state will continue for several more decades before a commonly agreed-upon set of socially integrated values and guidelines emerges. Without a sense of integrated community and belongingness, our cultural backdrop to violence will continue for some time to come.

Biological Theories

Many medical and behavioral scientific researchers have asked a fundamental question: Do abnormalities in biological structure and function result in violence? The answer is a complex and qualified "yes" in some, but not all, cases.

A first reasonable question is to ask whether there is any evidence to suggest that violence is genetic and inherited. The question is asked in part because some families are violent in succeeding generations and in part because some crimes are so heinous that most of us want to believe that there must have been some abnormality in the assailant at birth.

The research evidence to date is mixed. Some researchers such as Bouchard (1994) suggest that there is no known genetic basis for violence. Different violent persons committing the same crimes have no common genetic component. However, other investigators such as Guan Guo and his colleagues (Guo, Roettger, and Cai, 2008) report that the MAOA gene, the dopamine Transporter1 gene, and the dopamine D2 receptor gene in the presence of environmental stress may link adolescent delinquency to molecular genetic variants. Further genetic research is needed before conclusions may be drawn.

There is research evidence that documents that injury to the brain in the cortex or limbic system may result in violence. (See figure 5 in the first chapter.) Tumors, head injuries, viruses, birth defects, and exposure to lead are some of the events that may destroy the cortex and its cortical control centers that inhibit violent behavior. Similar injuries to the limbic system such as viruses, head injuries, and untreated psychological trauma may result in violence as well.

As seen in tables 1 and 2 in the first chapter, certain medical and psychiatric illnesses and conditions contain the potential for violence. In addition, certain bodily conditions may elevate the risk for violence. These include states of pain, hunger, sleep deprivation, excessive heat, overcrowding, and severe life-stress (e.g., divorce, foreclosure of mortgage, loss of job, terminal illness).

Four personality disorders – antisocial, borderline, narcissist, paranoid – have been at times associated with violence (American Psychiatric Association, 1994). The level of biological involvement in these personality disorders remains medically unclear. However, unlike some medical illnesses, there is no current evidence that these personality disorders and associated violence are necessarily beyond an individual's control. An antisocial person is one who is engaged in criminal activity toward person or property, is not governed by the prosocial values of society and is often morally depraved. The person with borderline disorder has intense mood swings from uncontrollable crying to intense oral hostility and rage. Some researchers believe that persons with borderline personality disorder may have a limbic system dysfunction. A narcissistic person is one who values oneself above all else and continuously wants one's own way. The individual with a paranoid personality is suspicious of most all persons and events. The world is seen as a hostile threat that requires constant vigilance to assure one's safety.

Some acts of violence appear biologically rooted and disrupt the domain of reasonable mastery. Given the nature of our care-providing work, we may see more biologically rooted violence than the general public. However, the total numbers of these cases is small and can in no way account for the total levels of present-day violence in our society.

The biological theories have their main impact on disruptions in the domain of mastery and to some extent meaningful purpose.

Sociological Theories

The sociological theorists of violence seek to explain what social environmental events in our daily lives may contribute to violence. The research has focused on poverty, inadequate schooling, discrimination, domestic violence, substance use, easily available weapons, and the media. Since these issues are routinely discussed in the media and are familiar subjects, they will be noted here briefly.

It has been known since the time of the Romans that poverty is highly correlated with crime and violence. In some cases, individuals without financial resources are forced to steal to feed, clothe, and shelter themselves. Some without adequate prosocial problem-solving skills earn a living by engaging in criminal behaviors, such as fencing stolen goods, fraud, or drug-trafficking. Still others who learn of the emphasis on material goods through the media break and enter, snatch purses, and commit robberies to obtain the material goods that they cannot legitimately afford.

Inadequate schooling compounds the problem of poverty in the postindustrial state. Knowledge and technology continue to become increasingly complex and those who drop out of school or who come from inadequate schools do not learn the socially sanctioned skills and educational skills necessary to obtain employment in the knowledge-based state. Schools without enough teachers, without enough books for each student, without adequate computer availability, and schools in physical disrepair do not adequately prepare children for earning a living in today's age.

Acts of discrimination are acts of hatred committed against innocent persons because of some aspect of their personhood. Age, race, ethnicity, creed, gender preference, and physical attributes are some of the more common areas of discrimination known to all of us. Every act of discrimination blocks some person or persons from equal access to basic civil rights and equal opportunities.

Domestic violence refers to violence committed by any family member or significant other toward any other family member or significant other. Such violence may involve grandparents, parents, children, extended family members and a variety of significant others who may be residing in the home. The abuse may include murder, physical and sexual abuse, nonverbal intimidation, verbal abuse, neglect, and/or mental torture. This is a serious problem encountered by health-care providers and is the subject matter of a later chapter.

Substance use is a serious national public health problem and includes the excessive use of alcohol and a variety of street drugs and prescription medications. Many times the substance use begins as a form of self-medication to soothe one's nerves but over time it becomes a physical addiction. Substance use impairs the individual's physical health and social well-being in terms of family disruptions, loss of employment, legal involvement, and similar. For caregivers, it is important to remember that substance use disinhibits the higher cortical-control centers in the brain and increases the potential for behavioral violence.

The presence of easily available weapons, especially those for purchase by children and adolescents in school playgrounds, has led to the increased use of firearms to settle conflicts over girlfriends, boyfriends, money, loss of face, and the like. Whereas in the past, the two parties might have had a fist fight, now each party is brandishing a weapon. So extensive is the problem, that innocent children now feel they have to arm themselves for protection, when they leave home. Legitimate gun holders who are licensed and use their weapons appropriately, such as for hunting, should be supported but society needs to address the presence of easily available weapons for children in our school neighborhoods.

Finally, the impact of the media needs to be addressed. There is an extensive national debate currently about whether video games increase the marksmanship of children. For some, it no doubt does but, as with the portrayal of violence in other media forms, most children who watch these violent episodes do not then become copycat assailants. There is a small subset of children who are unduly influenced by the violence in the media, including computer games. Further research is needed to identify these high-risk children. In the interim, society in general would benefit from parents engaging in media literacy with their children. Media literacy refers to educating the child as to the true and full meaning of what is being viewed. For example, after a scene of a violent car accident, the parent might discuss the importance of safe driving, the impact of the accident on the victim's health, the impact of the accident on the victim's family, and so forth. Discussions such as these teach children about the painful consequences of violence that are not portrayed in the media as it cuts to commercials.

In general, the sociological theories reflect disruptions in the domain of caring attachments and often reflect lack of empathy as a component.

Psychological Theories

The psychological theories refer to two main factors: the individual's coping skills and the individual's motivation for violent behavior. Coping skills refer to personal self-care skills, interpersonal skills, and academic skills. Self-care skills include sound health and nutrition practices, the importance of exercise, understanding the financial system, managing time, managing life-stress, and learning how to comfort oneself in personally difficult times. Interpersonal skills refer to an ability to interact well with others and include being able to identify our feeling states correctly, having empathy for others, expressing our needs tactfully, sharing with others, grieving, and using verbal-conflict resolution skills to solve interpersonal problems. Academic skills involve not only computer literacy but a strong foundation in all basic academic areas, including math, science, English, English composition, and history among other subjects.

The absence of these adequate coping skills, coupled with the absence of caring attachments, leaves the person without the prosocial skills and contacts to participate fully in the postindustrial state. In the face of this inability to participate in more socially acceptable ways, many turn to antisocial values. Their behavior is motivated by catharsis, anger, selfishness, self-indulgence, the enforcement of one's personal sense of justice, social acceptance in gangs, shame, and similar self-defeating motivational stances: see table 2.

The psychological theories result in disruptions in the domains of reasonable mastery and meaningful purpose.

This overview of the theories of human violence may be helpful for those of us in professional care-giving roles, if we link these theories to our discussion of the domains of good health. As we have noted, each grouping of theories implies the disruption of one of these basic domains that results in the increased risk for violence: the cultural theories with the destruction of caring attachments, the bio-

TABLE 2. Common Motivational Factors in Violence

Acceptance by Peers
Catharsis of Anger
Despair
Dominance of Others
Enforcement of Personal Sense of Justice
Excitement
Jealousy
Revenge
Selfishness
Shame
Status

logical theories with disruptions in mastery, the sociological theories with disruptions in attachments, and the psychological theories with shattered reasonable mastery and a prosocial meaningful purpose in life. An important message for caregivers is that, when encountering behavioral emergencies with potential for violence, we should look for small ways to restore a sense of attachment, a sense of reasonable mastery, and a sense of some meaningful purpose and we shall study how to do this in detail in later chapters.

For the moment, with these disruptions in mind, let us return to the opening vignette of the young man, Richard, who was hearing voices. Following the general safety guidelines thus far, we consider in advance what type of incident we are being called upon for assistance. This suspect/patient had psychosis, substance use, and, likely, untreated psychological trauma. Did we utilize the call log to see if we had encountered this young man before? If so, what information did we have? How did he present before? What was helpful then?

When the scene is surveyed, has anyone been hurt? Was anyone in immediate harm? Could those persons have been safely moved away? Did we come upon a weapon? Did we evaluate the suspect/patient for old brain-stem prominence? If we thought that to be the case, would it have made sense to give the individual time to calm down and think more clearly? There were warning signs of potential loss of control. He was ill-kempt, pacing, and furtive.

Our review of the theories of violence might also have been helpful here. He is living in an age of anomie; he has the medical issues of psychosis; he has the sociological issues of possible poverty and substance use; he is psychologically overwhelmed and frightened to the point that he cannot cope This information can be of use in efforts to help him. What medicine does he take? When was his last drink? What will help him to calm down? As we would expect from our review of the theories of violence, his domains of good health are also disrupted. Did he have any caring attachments that we could have called upon? Could we have made ourselves an interim attachment network? Could we have found some small way to restore his sense of mastery in the park? Perhaps, he could have told us how we could be of help. Perhaps, he would prefer to walk to the police car on his own. Perhaps, he would have liked a smoke break. Perhaps, he would rather choose to be diverted to an emergency room rather than to a jail cell. Finally, could we have aligned ourselves with his sense of meaningful purpose, which appears to be to protect him from a malevolent world? Could we have asked him how we could be of assistance in this regard?

These questions are not meant to second-guess the officers who responded to the call in difficult circumstances. It is meant only to illustrate how the information that we have reviewed in the past two chapters could be utilized to increase our ability to defuse potential behavioral violence in a safe way. When communication fails, violence follows.

Table 3 presents our basic general safety guidelines to which I have added the theories of violence that disrupt the three domains of good health. As noted, in the coming chapters specific safety guidelines for specific types of behavioral emergencies will be added to these general safety guidelines. Health-care providers will benefit from being familiar with both.

TABLE 3. Safety Guidelines

Think Medical or Psychiatric Illness
Think Call Log
Think Scene Surveillance
Think Old Brain Stem
Think Early Warning Signs
Think Theories of Violence

Having reviewed general assessment/risk management strategies and theories of human violence in the first section of this book, this next section focuses on four behavioral emergencies that are commonly encountered in practice: psychological trauma; domestic violence; psychosis/substance use/suicide; and youth violence/gang/street crime. First, we turn to psychological trauma. Many of the behavioral emergencies that we assist with are incidents that themselves have traumatized the person to whom we are providing care or service. Caregivers will want to be aware that these traumatized states in patients are also a potential second source of behavioral violence and to know why.

PART TWO

THE VIOLENT PERSON: COMMON CRITICAL INCIDENTS

THREE

Psychological Trauma

Never shall I forget those moments that murdered my God
And my soul and turned my dreams to dust.

—Elie Weisel

It was about 8:15 on a Tuesday morning. Evan sat quietly at home in his recliner chair and listened to soft music on the radio. As the words and melody to "Rain Drops Are Falling on My Head" began, he lurched out of his chair as if propelled by a cannon shot. He lay writhing on the floor, his pulse was over 140, his blood pressure was 175/110. His body was shaking, his teeth chattering, and his bones registering the chill of death, as if he had been left for hours in the cold snows of winter. He gasped for breath. He was crying. He was in sheer terror and inconsolable agony. His dark night of the soul had once again returned.

Raindrops. Raindrops? Raindrops on a bright sunny morning in late summer in New York City? How could that be?

But it was true. There were raindrops. Human raindrops. Persons who had elected to jump from eighty to one hundred floors above to their deaths below rather than burn in the Twin Towers inferno that engulfed them all. Many hoped that they would die of a heart attack on the way down. They called home on cell phones to say one last good-bye to loved ones, then to say a small prayer, and then finally to jump into the abyss.

As a first responder nurse, Evan knew that he could not break these falls because the force of their impact would kill him as well. Thus, he had to stand there helplessly. Many of these precious raindrops did not have fatal heart attacks on the way down but were alive and killed instantly on impact. Evan witnessed the final agonizing screams of death, crushed skulls, broken limbs, and spattered pools of blood, brains, and flesh.

Cell phones rang as loved ones called back for just one last moment together. These cold human raindrops of death had become Evan's dark night of the soul.

Evan has a serious medical condition known as *posttraumatic stress disorder* (PTSD). He is not alone. Many persons have this medical condition. It evolves from untreated psychological trauma.

Psychological trauma is an individual's response to a life-threatening situation, over which the individual has no control, no matter how hard the person tries. Natural and man-made disasters; incineration of buildings; rail, aircraft, and motor-vehicle accidents may all cause psychological trauma. In addition, acts of human-perpetrated violence may do so as well. If psychological trauma is not treated, it becomes PTSD. If PTSD is not treated, the victim will carry the scars of this medical condition to the grave.

Psychological trauma and untreated PTSD are common components in behavioral emergencies. These can come about in several ways. First, the emergency itself may be in response to incidents that can traumatize in and of themselves, such as first psychotic episodes or domestic violence. Here the events themselves may have victimized the individuals involved. Second, the present behavioral emergency that in itself is not necessarily traumatic may create psychological trauma in some predisposed individuals. A person of color at home who has been robbed may become traumatized by derogatory comments by a person at work, as the person remembers being mistreated by the robbers. Third, the present behavioral emergency may be a symbolic reminder of other posttraumatic events and the individual who may not be presently injured may still experience the thoughts, feelings and behaviors of the similar, earlier event. For example, some health-care providers responded to a minor car accident where the sole, uninjured, female victim was running around the car proclaiming that her son was dead. There was no body of her son at the scene. However, the present accident reminded her of a fatal accident some years before that had claimed the life of her son. Finally, we health-care providers may become victims of psychological trauma ourselves, if we have been direct victims ourselves, if we witness and care for others who have been mangled in all sorts of ways, and/or if they recount what has happened to them.

The suffering of the victims of psychological trauma and PTSD is painful for us care-providers to observe and assist with. However, there is second and ominous implication as well. Untreated psychological trauma and PTSD may lead the victim to become violent in his or her own right at a later point in time. We who respond onsite in a specific critical incident may not know that the present victim has a past trauma history and may be functioning with old brain-stem prominence. Therefore, it is important that we recognize trauma when we see it and know how to respond to such victims to enhance safety and keep the behavioral emergency from erupting into violence.

Identify and caring for victims of psychological trauma is the first of the specific assessment/risk management strategies that we want to become familiar with in this second part of the book.

The Nature of Psychological Trauma and Posttraumatic Stress Disorder (PTSD)

Psychological trauma is a person's physical and psychological response to having experienced, witnessed, or been confronted with events that involve actual or threatened death, serious injury, or threat to physical integrity of self or others (American Psychiatric Association, 1994). It must involve intense fear, helplessness, or horror, such that any adult would be frightened. In children this intense fear may manifest itself in disorganized or agitated behavior. As we noted above, natural and man-made disasters, major technological failures that claim lives, combat, and the many forms of human-perpetrated violence are all potentially traumatizing events in that they are life-threatening and we as individuals have no control over these events, no matter how hard we try.

Any of us may become a victim of psychological trauma in one of three ways. The first is by direct act in which we are attacked, threatened, or directly harmed. The second way is by witnessing these traumatic situations impacting on others. We may be direct witnesses to the incident or, as frequently happens to caregivers, witnesses to the incident's impact and its aftermath on the patient victims that we care for. The third way is through vicarious traumatization. This refers to the care-provider, family member, neighbor, or others who develop psychological trauma, by listening to the victim's recounting of the traumatic crisis.

Domains of Good Health

Traumatic events may disrupt any of the three domains of good health and result in impaired functioning in attachments, reasonable mastery, or meaningful purpose.

Attachments. First, caring attachments may be torn apart. This may be due to the actual deaths and separations of loved ones and/or disruptions in community life. In addition, the victim may perceive the world as not safe and other persons as potential assailants. This latter fear is especially common in human-perpetrated violence and victims withdraw from daily life activity to some perceived safe environment.

The loss of caring attachments is further compounded by the behavior of nonvictims. Traumatic incidents again teach how tenuous our links are to Mother Earth. To provide ourselves with the illusion of some control, we blame the victims for their predicaments. Instead of identifying them as being the wrong person in the wrong place, we blame them for being victims of natural disasters or criminal behavior. "If they hadn't been on the beach, they would not have been swept away in the Tsunami." "If she didn't wear shorts, she wouldn't have been raped." "If he hadn't gone across the city common at dusk, he wouldn't have been mugged." Statements such as these are meant to provide nonvictims with the illusion of control. The implication is that the nonvictims would not be as foolish a risk-taker as the victims and, thus, would be saved from harm. The problem, of course, is that it *is* an illusion and contains no guarantee of safety. The tragedy here is that, at the moment when victims most need caring attachments, those potential caring attachments have pulled away in an opposite direction.

Mastery. The loss of reasonable mastery in traumatic events is self-evident. By definition, these are crises beyond the control of the victims. People with reasonable mastery skills are suddenly overwhelmed. They may respond in any number of ways. They may flee in panic, they may freeze in terror, they may develop learned helplessness, they may become super-vigilant about the smallest of details to prevent a recurrence. They may use drugs or alcohol to self-medicate the terror and chaos. None of these strategies is effective in addressing the crisis but such disrupted mastery behavior may last for hours, days, or years. Each of us has a psychological boundary about ourselves that reinforces our sense of control. It is about a foot in distance and people need permission to come closer inside that psychological boundary. Parents, children, close friends may enter but not strangers. When a traumatic event occurs, the victim's sense of boundaries is torn down and the victim feels helpless in the onslaught of forces beyond the victim's control. It is a very frightening feeling.

Meaningful Purpose. When we got up this morning, each of us made some assumptions about the world around us. We assumed that the world was orderly, safe, reasonably predictable, and worthy of our investing energy in it. For victims of violence these assumptions are often shattered by the nature of the traumatic event. The world does not seem orderly, safe, and predictable after the onset of a sudden, violent incident and it certainly does not feel to victims that they want to remain or become a part of it.

Victims physically and psychologically withdraw. When careproviders arrive to assist, the victim's psychological boundaries for safety have been shattered. The victims are often experiencing the raw, brunt force of the crises and they may well be functioning with old brain-stem prominence. In these cases, they may need health care assistance to reestablish cortical control.

Symptoms of Psychological Trauma and PTSD

As with any medical condition, psychological trauma and its untreated counterpart, PTSD, have signs or symptoms that the mind and body are not functioning properly. When a crisis erupts, certain biological chemicals in the victims are activated to protect the victims but they may also result in trauma/PTSD symptoms.

Our nervous system is a series of nerve fibers joined together by small balloon-like vesicles known as *synaptic gaps:* see figure 1. These gaps contain chemicals that are known as *neurotransmitters.* These neurotransmitters prepare us so that we are best able to cope with the crisis at hand. Common neurotransmitters include adrenalin, which becomes epinephrine in the body and norepinephrine in the brain; and cortisol, serotonin, and the endorphins.

FIGURE 1. The Synaptic Gap

(with Neurotransmitters)

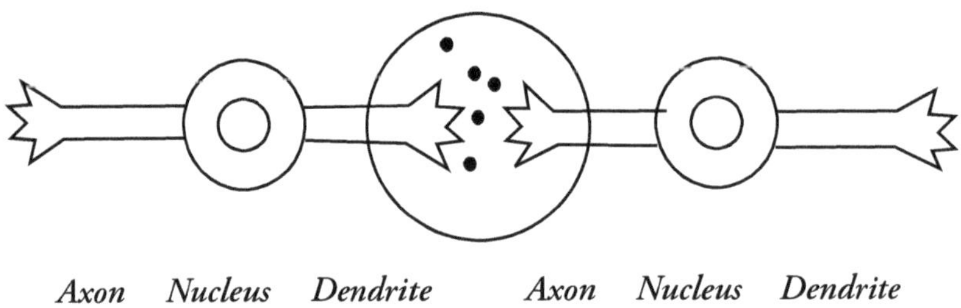

Adrenalin is activated instantly and causes the individual to become immediately attentive. As epinephrine in the body, adrenalin enervates the heart, lungs, and muscles to work effectively and efficiently. Epinephrine dilates pupils, so that potential victims see more clearly and it dampens down bodily functions that are not necessary for immediate survival, such as digestion. Cortisol is released and this provides the individual with increased sources of energy and blood clotting ability to survive wounds.

In the brain, adrenalin becomes norepinephrine and rivets the person's attention to the crisis at hand.

Two additional chemicals are at work in the brain during a crisis. Serotonin, a chemical that normally makes us feel good, is utilized as a catalyst in a crisis to make norepinephrine function more efficiently. Chemicals called endorphins which also normally make us feel good, act as analgesics to deaden pain in a crisis. Various combinations of these neurotransmitters result in the trauma symptoms noted in table 1.

TABLE 1. Symptoms of Psychological Trauma and Posttraumatic Stress Disorder

Physical Symptoms	Hypervigilance Exaggerated Startle Response Difficulty Sleeping Difficulty with Concentration, Memory Mood Irritability – Especially Anger and Depression
Intrusive Symptoms	Recurring, Distressing Recollections (Thoughts, Memories, Dreams, Nightmares, Flashbacks) Physical or Psychological Distress at an Event That Symbolizes the Trauma Grief or Survivor Guilt
Avoidant Symptoms	Avoiding Specific Thoughts, Feelings, Activities or Situations Diminished Interest in Significant Activities Restricted Range of Emotions (Numbness)

The physical symptoms are primarily the result of adrenalin and cortisol in the body. Hypervigilance, exaggerated startle response, difficulty sleeping and concentrating, and angry outbursts reflect the full flow of adrenalin in the victim. It is nature's way of providing the victim every opportunity for survival.

The intrusive symptoms are primarily memories of the event and are thought to be present because of adrenalin and the endorphins being in the brain. The victim keeps reviewing the tragedy day and night in dreams, recollections, nightmares, and the like. Similarly, symbolic reminders of the situation can result in revisiting traumatic events in memory. For example, the ex-combat soldier at home who hears a bus backfire and is reminded of the sounds of artillery shells in war. Finally, grief and survivor-guilt are included as intrusive memories because the grieving survivor is always thinking of those who died in the traumatic event. Intrusive memories appear to be the brain's method of healing itself. It is saying to the victim: review what has happened so that you will be better prepared next time, should it ever happen again. However, these memories are very painful and many victims try to put them out of their minds through various methods of distraction.

The avoidant symptoms are fundamentally symptoms of withdrawal from life. Adrenalin and serotonin appear to have been depleted or used up, a state that leaves the victim weary and depressed. The intrusive memories of the event are a further burden. In these circumstances many victims immediately withdraw from the scene of the traumatic incident and over time withdraw from a whole range of activities in life that were previously of interest. Emotions become restricted. The person is never really happy, never really excited about life, but instead develops a chronic sense of mild to moderate depression. If the trauma/PTSD is not treated, these sufferings will last until death.

Stages of Psychological Trauma and PTSD

Figure 2 outlines the stages or phases that victims of psychological trauma and PTSD may go through. The traumatic event occurs and acute psychological distress follows immediately. The distress is manifested by disruptions in the three domains of good health and/or by the presence of any of the trauma symptoms. Victims average about thirty days to recover and restore some semblance of normal daily living. This timeframe is based on the amount of time the average victim needs to recover. Traumatic events differ in their severity and people differ widely in their coping skills, so there are understandable individual differences with this time span.

FIGURE 2. Stages in Psychological Trauma and Posttraumatic Stress Disorder

The Traumatic Event

↓

Acute Distress

↓

Posttraumatic Stress Disorder

↓

Acute PTSD

↓

Chronic PTSD

↓

Delayed Onset PTSD

If the victim is still experiencing disruptions in the health domains and/or the presence of symptoms on the thirty-first day, the person develops the medical condition known as posttraumatic stress disorder (PTSD). There are three types of PTSD. The first is acute PTSD, which is defined as disruptions in the domains of good health and/ or the presence of trauma symptoms that occurred during the acute distress period and continue for as long as the next three months.

If the symptoms continue four months or beyond after the acute distress phase, the victim has developed chronic PTSD with domain disruptions and/or trauma symptoms that will last until death in the absence of treatment. In these chronic PTSD cases, it is not uncommon for a subsequent acute traumatic stress situation to serve as symbolic stimulus or reminder for the recall of memories originally associated with the first traumatic incident.

The last form of PTSD is known as delayed onset PTSD. In these cases, a victim was originally distressed by the event during the acute distress phase but seemed to quickly return to normal daily living. At some point after six months of normal daily routines, the health domain disruptions and/or trauma symptomatology originally associated with the event return in full, vivid, frightening recall. This latent recall is precipitated by a symbolic reminder or by a major loss. All traumatic incidents involve loss such as the loss of physical integrity in battering, the loss of free choice in rape, or the loss of innocence in the world in combat. In this way, loss through death, failing senses, financial reversal, and similar events may result in the return of intrusive memories.

Special Issues in Psychological Trauma and PTSD

There are certain behavioral issues that are frequently found in trauma and that may complicate the victims' lives and recoveries. These include self-medication, dissociation, the repetition compulsion, unresolved grief, and, regrettably, subsequent victim-perpetrated violence.

Self-medication

If one were to go onto hospital wards where victims of psychological trauma were being treated, the patients' charts would likely contain two diagnoses. The first, not surprisingly, would be untreated PTSD. The second diagnosis, however, would be substance use disorder. This would be true in a great many cases. The medical charts of cardiac or cancer patients would not carry frequent diagnoses of co-occurring substance use disorders.

TABLE 2. Substance Use and the Self-medication Hypothesis

Substance	*Type of Psychological Distress*
Amphetamines Cocaine	Depression
Alcohol Barbiturates	Anxiety
Opiates	Anger

When individuals are victims of violence, they are terrified. They experience disruptions in the domains of good health and the symptoms of trauma and PTSD, as we have seen. Most commonly, they do not realize that they are victims of psychological trauma and they do not realize that they have a diagnosable medical condition for which there is treatment. In their lack of understanding, they turn to drugs or alcohol to calm their nerves and reduce their intense emotional distress.

Psychiatrist Edward Khantzian (1997) noticed that people who abused substances had a drug of choice, if they had the money to buy it. He also noticed that certain favorite drugs of choice were being used to medicate certain types of feelings. Table 2 presents a brief summary of his findings.

Persons using amphetamines and crack/cocaine were self-medicating depression. Persons using alcohol or barbiturates were medicating anxiety, and persons using the various types of opiates (e.g., oxycontin) were self-medicating states of anger and rage. A good many of the self-medicating patients that he observed had trauma histories, so one could speculate that in some cases the feeling states that they were self-medicating, were feelings that came about as a result of their traumatic incidents.

This self-medication information may be of assistance to health-care providers who are asked to respond to an emergency in which substance use or a history of substance use are present. Knowing the drug of choice will tell you something about the psychology of your victim and what mood states you might expect, especially if withdrawal is in progress.

Dissociation

When a person is confronted with a life-or-death situation, the person's brain has the remarkable capacity to put out of immediate mental presence all information that is not necessary for survival which, if considered, might distract the person and result in death. If three comrades are in a foxhole in combat and take a direct hit so that only one survives, the survivor's brain will put all unnecessary information aside so that that soldier can focus on survival. The brain will not become preoccupied with the deaths of comrades and increase the risk of the soldier's own death.

This process is known as dissociation and the information that is not needed for survival is temporarily put aside in the person's memory. This is called a dissociated memory. When the crisis has past, this dissociated memory returns to the person's consciousness and is known as a *flashback.* Although these memories are very vivid, they seem to follow the rules of normal memory (McNally, 2003). The victim's review of the dissociated material appears to be the brain's way of reviewing the material to see if anything can be learned in case such a crisis should ever happen again. Since these memories are unpleasant, many victims find some way to distract themselves from these unpleasant thoughts, as we have noted, and in doing so lay the groundwork for the trauma to remain untreated. Victims of combat and rape are the victims most likely to experience dissociative episodes. Flashbacks are most likely to be tripped off by symbolic reminders or by losses.

The Repetition Compulsion

One of the continuing mysteries of psychological trauma is a phenomenon known as the repetition compulsion. One would think that, if you were a victim of violence, that you would move as far away as possible to safety and most victims do. Yet, there is a small group of victims who go back into harm's way, when there is no reason to do so.

I have seen this frequently in health care. Some health-care providers are always in the middle of patient assaults. At first, one reviews the safety procedures of nonviolent self-defense approaches to be sure that staff members are technically skilled. When one is assured of this competence, then one must look for some other explanation for this phenomenon. Certain theorists believe the repetition compulsion is an attempt to learn better mastery skills for better protection in the future (e.g., the sexual abuse victim who engages in prostitution). Other scientists are studying various possible biological explanations for this phenomenon. In any case, the so-called frequent flyers that health-care providers encounter may be examples of persons with repetition compulsions.

Unresolved Grief

As we have noted, all trauma involves loss of some form. Your family abuses you or walks out on you. Your innocent children are murdered in drive-by gang shootings. Your experiences of incest or sexual abuse leave you feeling like damaged goods. The sexual abuse among ministers challenges your religious faith. If nothing else, human-perpetrated violence shatters your innocence of the world. Since many victims are ashamed of what has befallen them and society's nonvictims do not want to hear about such things, the victim's grief often remains unspoken, unshared, and unresolved.

Although there are several models for understanding grieving, perhaps the most common one is the five-step model of Kübler-Ross (1997). Dr. Kübler-Ross did her studies on patients who were dying, but it turns out that steps for grieving death are similar for any loss (e.g., divorce, not being promoted, financial loss). In Dr. Kübler-Ross's model the first step is denial in which the person refuses to accept the facts of what has happened. For example, a patient might protest that the laboratory tests suggesting cancer are really someone else's laboratory reports. The second step is one of anger. The person facing the loss becomes very angry about the loss and the person's anger can be displaced or placed on others who are innocent bystanders to the loss. In the third step, the person bargains with God, with the doctors, with the powers to be in any individual case to mitigate the loss somehow. The person bargains to have it be less severe or to be put off for some time. In step four the person becomes really depressed as the weight of the loss begins to sink in. Finally, in time, in step five the person becomes resigned to one's fate. Not all people go through all five steps or go through them in the most common sequence outlined here but grieving is an important part of life and must be addressed.

If a person is not fully grieving a loss that is severe or that is protracted over time, that person may develop clinical depression and the need for antidepressant medications. If left untreated, the person may become suicidal. Recent medical research suggests that, at least in some cases, suicide may be a biologically based medical condition. Every year in this country, suicides are about one percent of the population and this has basically not wavered since the Civil War, when medical statistics in our country started to be recorded. In addition, recent research on persons who had completed suicide in Scandinavia showed the brains of these persons to have serious serotonin depletion. This suggests a possible biological basis for suicide in that these individuals were born with less serotonin than normal or that somehow it was used up more quickly than normal and additional research is now being undertaken (Mann, 2003).

Behavioral emergencies by definition imply some sort of loss in health and functioning and caregivers will do well to pay attention to the presence of unresolved grief. One would want to be especially aware of a patient or family member in the second step, that of anger, since that anger in the person's grief may be misdirected in violent ways toward the team that is there to help.

Violence by Victims

An important reason for identifying and treating trauma in behavioral emergency victims is that these early interventions may mitigate and prevent the use of violence at a later time by the patient who is currently the trauma victim being treated. In many cases, victims of untreated trauma and PTSD go on to become violent. Children sexually abused as children have gone on to rape. Children who have been battered as children have grown up to batter others. There are many types of examples of this phenomenon.

Why would they do this, especially when they know how painful it is to be the victim? There are several possible paths toward this end. One, which we just examined, is the anger and depression over what has happened. If the victim's grief for each incident is unresolved, then that anger may surface and others may be victimized. Some victims have learned that violence works, so they use violence as a mode of solving problems. Others want revenge to settle old scores. For still others, the use of substances may have disinhibited the cortical control centers in the brain leading to violence. Finally, as we shall see in the section below, the experience of psychological trauma may change the biology of the brain of the trauma victim, so that the victim is hard-wired to see the world as malevolent and to act accordingly on that perception.

Psychological Trauma and Changes in the Brain

Mentioned in passing earlier in the chapter is the role of neurotransmitters in the development of the symptoms of psychological trauma and PTSD. This section considers two additional changes that are possible in brain functioning in traumatic stress. One is in the prefrontal cortex (See figure 5, chapter 1) called Broca's Area and the other is in the limbic system. Both have serious implications for the work of health-care providers.

Broca's Area is found in the left side of the prefrontal cortex and permits the person to tell others what is happening and what they are feeling. Under very severe stress, when old brain-stem functioning is prominent, a person's Broca's Area may temporarily shut down. The person becomes mute and is unable to communicate orally. The person is immobilized and in a state of psychological shock. This state may last as long as several hours and subsides when the immediate overwhelming life-stress has passed.

FIGURE 3. The Limbic System

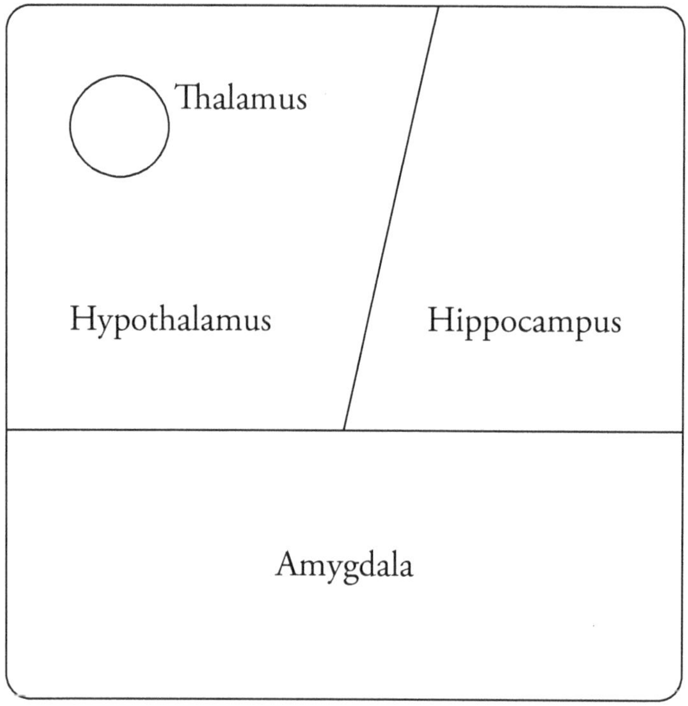

Our second area of inquiry is the limbic system. Figure 3 presents a drawing of the limbic system that is neither anatomically precise nor drawn to scale. In the diagram, the amygdala is that part of the limbic system where emotions are registered in the brain. Feelings of anger, sadness, contentment, excitement and so forth all register here on their way to the cortex. The hippocampus is the part of the limbic system that allows the person to label what he or she is feeling. The thalamus is a relay station for some of the body's sense pathways and sends these sense messages to the cortex. The hypothalamus is the highest center of integration for many visceral processes and, for our purposes here, is the engine that makes the limbic system work smoothly.

Recent research has found that in untreated PTSD victims, the hippocampus has atrophied, that is, its cells have died. Without hippocampal language the victim is unable to tell us how he or she is feeling. (In a Broca's Area shutdown, victims would be completely mute.) Hippocampal victims, however, can describe the events, the sequence, and so forth, but they are unable to label their psychological distress. There is some recent research suggesting that an atrophied hippocampus may regenerate itself but further study is needed.

In addition, early and prolonged stress in children results in increased adrenalin for hypervigilance, increased cortisol for the energy to be able to defend oneself, an increase in vasopressin that results in hostility and irritability, a decrease in serotonin resulting in less behavioral control, and a decrease in oxytocin that results in fewer caring, faithful relationships. Many of these changes occur in the limbic system (Teicher, Andersen, Polcari, Anderson, and Navalta, 2002). Additional research on the impact of trauma on the brains of children has shown brain volume to be smaller with fewer language skills and lowered serotonin, which may result in depression and impulsive aggression (Creeden, 2005; Finklehor and Jones, 2006). These early research findings demonstrate clearly that psychological trauma is not good for one's health and normal functioning.

These findings also suggest that severe traumatic stress modifies the brain to live in what it perceives as a malevolent world. The changes in brain neurochemistry result in suspiciousness, paranoia, and hypervigilance that lead to social isolation, depression, and lifelong medical problems such as diabetes and cardiovascular disease. The brain becomes modified for survival in the jungle and it is important for all caregivers to remember that they may be perceived as part of the jungle, when they first arrive onsite to provide care. (For further study of psychological trauma and PTSD, see Flannery [2004] and Herman [1992].)

Specific Safety Guidelines for Addressing Psychological Trauma Victims

To understand how best to approach trauma victims safely, we need to consider a person's sense of psychological self. As we have noted, each of us has a psychological boundary of about twelve inches about us and no one is permitted within that psychological boundary without our permission. When someone hits us, we feel violated because our psychological space has been intruded upon, in addition to the physical assault itself. If you want to see the power of this phenomenon, ask a colleague to stand in the middle of the room. Tell the person that you will not touch or harm him or her and that you will walk toward your colleague. When you get within the twelve-inch range, the person will move away from you.

When you are a trauma victim, this psychological boundary is shattered. The victim feels helpless, defenseless, and exposed to continuing violence. Providers who come to help may be seen as the enemy returning once again. Unless the victim is in an immediate, dire medical, life-threatening situation, stay at a distance from the victim whom you think may also be a trauma victim. State who you are, where you are, and why you are there. Repeat this until you know that the victim clearly understands this. This process begins to help the victim establish his or her boundaries. Ask in advance if you may have permission to move within what would be the normal twelve-inch boundary. Do not enter until you are given permission. Ask repeatedly until you are given that permission. State in advance what intervention you are going to employ and explain slowly how it will work. Ask for permission to do this. If you have a mixed-gender team, ask if there is any gender preference. Restore mastery by asking the patient to help you in some fashion. Begin to restore attachments by asking whom to notify. Begin to explore why this incident happened and what meaning it has in the person's life.

If you come upon a patient who is dissociating and having flashbacks, gently tell the patient who he or she is, who you are, and describe the immediate environment in some detail. Ground the patient in the here and now. As the patient becomes aware of the surroundings, explain to the patient that he or she was dissociating but that he or she is safe.

Let us return to Evan, the nurse in the vignette in this chapter. One can see now that he was suffering from untreated PTSD. When he had his flashbacks, he was experiencing physical and intrusive trauma symptoms. He tried to avoid these by not thinking about the Twin Towers. He appears to have gone back to work, a factor indicating that some level of mastery has been restored. We are not told of his attachments and, thus, are not able to assess for disruptions in this domain. However, it is clear that he has not been able to make meaning of the dark night of his soul. As we provide care, let us consider two final questions: What possible permanent changes may be taking place in his limbic system because of his untreated PTSD? Will he in time come to view the world as malevolent?

Table 3 presents both the general and specific safety guidelines that we have reviewed thus far.

TABLE 3. Safety Guidelines

- *Think Medical and Psychiatric Illness*
- *Think Call Log*
- *Think Scene Surveillance*
- *Think Old Brain Stem*
- *Think Early Warning Signs*
- *Think Theories of Violence*
- *Think Psychological Trauma*

We turn our attention next to another specific behavioral emergency that is itself all too common: domestic violence.

FOUR

Domestic Violence

Loneliness and the feeling of being unwanted
is the most terrible poverty.

—Mother Teresa

The pain in her rewired jaw was agonizing, even with pain medication, and her soul was in even more intense pain. Joanne was without hope and yet it had always been hope that had enabled her to carry on.

As she lay in her hospital bed, she thought back to her childhood: an alcoholic father, a mother who had psychologically withdrawn into the woodwork, two younger siblings who were always fighting. It was a dysfunctional family by any standard. When her father had been drunk, he beat them all and repeatedly raped her. He had told her that he would rape and beat her even more, if she ever shed a tear. She never shed a tear. The incest had stopped when she had turned fifteen and had threatened to call the police.

But what man would want her now? She was modestly attractive but with a nose that she thought too large. She had good parenting skills, skills that her father had forced her to learn when her mother abdicated being a parent. Yet, as her father continuously reminded her, she was sexually damaged goods. Who would want her? Hope for a better future, coupled with youthful idealism, kept her going.

When William walked into her life, her heart leapt with a joy that she had never known. For the first time in her life she experienced happiness. She had dreams for a future. She believed in God again. William had had an alcoholic parent, too, but that was behind them now. She thought of the words of Anne Frank – surely these pitiful days will come to an end.

Yet, now, eight years into her marriage, terror was her daily companion. William had proved to be an angry alcoholic like his father. William was even more violent than her own father had been. Forced, humiliating group sex and sex with animals were regularly interspersed with physical abuse of all types from cattle prods to cigarette burns to scalding acids. Anything handy! Last night he had slashed her face with a knife and had broken her now rewired jaw with a hammer.

What had begun in dreams had ended in ashes. God had died. Hope had died. Her heart had broken for the final time.

These pitiful days had not come to an end.

"Home sweet home." "Home is where the heart is." "Family values are best." Our culture is full of such aphorisms about the central role of home and family as a refuge from the slings and arrows of the larger world, as a place of comfort and support, as a source of love.

Although there are obviously many happy homes, such is not always the case. Sadly, research has demonstrated that home is actually one of the most violent institutions in contemporary society, the place where most of us are likely to encounter any harm that may befall us. Domestic violence includes murder, torture, all forms of physical and sexual abuse, nonverbal intimidation (threats with objects rather than words), verbal abuse, and, in the case of children, abandonment and neglect. This violence frequently results in psychological trauma as well.

Domestic violence occurs in homes to be sure but spills out into the community as assailants pursue their family members to worksites, hospital emergency rooms, nursing homes, and even church picnics. Domestic violence is found in both men and women and in all agcs, all races, all creeds, all ethnic groups, and all social classes. Health-care providers should consider every domestic violence call to be one of potential danger.

Domestic violence leaves raw wounds. The three domains of good health are crushed. Caring attachments may be destroyed literally and are revealed to be at least as empty and nonsupportive. Violence leaves victims angry, embarrassed, frightened, depressed, suspicious of others, and reticent to trust anyone. Mastery has been disrupted because verbal conflict resolutions have failed to find nonviolent solutions to family problems and a meaningful purpose in family life, a community of caring and affection, has been reduced to ashes.

Abraham Lincoln once wrote that defeat strikes the young the hardest because they least expect it and the young in domestic violence situations, whether direct victims or victim witnesses, are especially vulnerable. The care and protection that should be freely given by their adult caregivers are either not provided adequately or are absent altogether.

In the chapter we shall examine people's inhumanity to one another. Caregivers will want to consider the various possible dynamics of what has transpired before the call for assistance is received. Who does these things? Why do they do them? What is the likely impact on those whom we are asked to assist? Although verbal abuse and nonverbal intimidation are extensive and very frightening in their own right, in the interests of space we shall focus on the more severe extremes of domestic violence: the sexual abuse of children and adult family members, and the physical abuse, torture, and murder of both children and adult members of the household.

The General Nature of Domestic Violence

Domestic violence is defined formally as any unwanted physical, sexual, or other unwanted contact, as well as verbal abuse, nonverbal intimidation, neglect, or abandonment by one family member or significant other toward another family member or significant other. It is true for heterosexual and homosexual couples and for those living together.

Let us begin by examining some common misunderstandings of assailants and victims. Persons who are battered are not masochistic; they are not seeking to be punished and they don't enjoy it. Battery occurs across all social classes including the very wealthy, so it is not necessarily a function of poverty. Batterers are not necessarily life's losers who cannot cope with life in general. Many are highly skilled craftsmen and professionals. Batterers are not violent in all of their relationships. They may behave well at work and be torturous at home. Many young people believe that the battering on dates will stop when they are married. It will not. Battering takes on a life of its own and increases in severity and frequency over time. Substance use makes battering worse because the cortical control centers of the brain are disinhibited, as we have seen. Finally, some nonbattering parents believe it is better for the children to stay with the batterers, so that the children have two parents. What is being overlooked in these cases is that the children may be traumatized by the family's violence and resort to such violence in their own lives, when they become adults later on.

In general, men and women who batter come from dysfunctional families, have themselves been personally victimized as children, have a substance use disorder, and many feel especially entitled. The entitled ones treat family members as if they were their own personal property. It is a deadly mix of dysfunctional behaviors with often horrific results, as the chapter example of Joanne illustrates.

The Nature of Sexual Abuse

Sexual abuse occurs when one person forces sexual intimacy of some form on a non-consenting partner. In domestic-violence contexts in the home, any female or male family, member or significant other, can perpetrate this violence on any other family member or significant other, regardless of age or formal role in the family structure. Nonconsent means the person consciously refuses consent, is without the capacity to give consent (e.g., date-rape drugs), or has not reached the age of reason to give consent.

Adult Sexual Abuse

Sexual abuse occurs in marriage when one spouse forces the other unwilling partner to engage in some normal or deviant sexual activity. D.E. H. Russell (1990) was the first to document this ugly form of human degradation between spouses. Forced rape in marriage may include practices such as sadomasochistic behavior, forced group sex, objects placed in the vagina, beatings, cigarette burns, use of cattle prods, urinating on a person, forced sex with animals, verbal degradation, and similar "sexual" practices.

Child Sexual Abuse

Similarly, degrading forms of sexual abuse may occur between parents and children, siblings, grandparents and grandchildren, or other combination that is biologically possible. The most common form of child sexual abuse is incest, which is defined as the rape or other form of sexual abuse of one's child, stepchild, or relative. The child who should be protected is exploited.

There are common characteristics in incest cases. It usually occurs between the ages of four and twelve years; it occurs more than once; and it stops around age fifteen, when the victim threatens to tell someone in authority or runs away. Child sexual abuse can be perpetrated by either parent gender in all possible combinations of parent/child gender relationships.

Family Incest Dynamics. Denise J. Gelinas (1983) was among the first to document how incest develops in many families. The father feels entitled. He is tyrannical and frequently addicted to alcohol or drugs. He comes from a dysfunctional family where he was abandoned, abused, and/or deprived. One of his great fears is that of being abandoned again. This father marries a woman who also has a victim-abuse history and was "parentified" as a child. Being parentified means that a parent has psychologically withdrawn from the family unit and one of the children is required to take on the parenting responsibilities for the siblings in the family. His wife was parentified and required to rear her siblings and do the housework in her adolescent years. As a teenager, before marriage, his wife, felt unloved but she was drawn to men with the need to be taken care of. Hence, the needs of both emerged as the foundation for a less than optimal marriage.

These two young adults marry and the marriage proceeds moderately well until the birth of the second child. At that point, the parentified wife can no longer cope with child rearing responsibilities, feels overwhelmed, and emotionally withdraws from the family as her own parent had. The father now fears being abandoned and rejected as he was in his family of origin and reaches out for his daughter sexually. The seduction is usually gradual in steps and frequently the daughter is showered with gifts and attention. Their daughter becomes parentified and the cycle starts again.

This form of sexual license assumed by the parent may be equally assumed by grandparents, aunts, uncles, cousins, and siblings. In addition, some extended families have pedophiles within their ranks and these pedophiles prey on the family unit's children in additionally deviant ways.

The Nature of Physical Abuse

Physical abuse in homes is frequent. Parents attack each other, parents attack their children, parents attack their parents, children attack their parents, children attack their siblings. If this were not enough, other family members such as aunts and uncles may also become violent. Strauss and Gelles (1992) have provided the most thorough documentation to date of this legacy of shame.

Adult Physical Abuse

As with child incest, battering by adult partners also appears to follow a pattern. Most of the abuse occurs between 8:00 and 11:30 P.M. on weekends or holidays, twelve hours after the assailant has begun drinking. Most of the abuse occurs in the kitchen. In those cases that culminate in murder, the murder takes place in the bedroom where there is only one exit.

Weapons vary. The hairbrush is the most common instrument but other weapons have also included guns, cattle prods, baseball bats, belts, scissors, chains, hot water, acid, bleach, bricks, coat hangers, tools, cigarette burns. Injuries may be severe and may include cuts and lacerations, broken bones, dislocated spines, lost teeth, damage to internal organs, and, in some instances, paralysis.

The Cycle of Violence. This spousal abuse often follows a cycle of violence first documented by L. Walker (2000). Table 1 outlines the three-step cycle. The first stage is the tension-building phase in which the spouse and every family member know that the violence is building and will erupt at some point. Many assailants have a cycle (weekly, monthly, every third month, and so forth), so that families learn to assess the increases in tension in the home. The second stage is the inevitable outburst in which the assailant behaves abusively, until his or her strength runs out. The third phase is the contrition phase in which the assailant promises never to do it again, sends candy and flowers, has his or her parent call

TABLE 1. The Cycle of Domestic Violence

1. *The Tension-Building Phase*
2. *The Inevitable Outburst Phase*
3. *The Contrition Phase*

to make amends. Since no one wants to be battered, when the crisis has passed and the spouse is contrite, many a battered victim returns to the partner and the cycle starts again.

The contrition phase has been a serious issue for police and the justice system. Victims who swore out complaints the night of the assault would come to court during the contrition phase and ask that all charges be dropped. The legal community responded to this by passing laws that required police to both arrest and prosecute the assailants, regardless of the victim's wishes. It was thought that this approach would reduce domestic violence and, in many instances it has. However, recent research (Mills, 2003) has shown that it reduces domestic violence mainly in middle- and upper-middle-class families where the assailants face the loss of public face. In lower-class families, the research demonstrates that arresting and prosecuting the assailant results in worse violence, when the assailant is released. Additional research is needed to develop strategies to stop domestic violence in the lower classes.

Why Don't the Victims Leave? Given that the victim is being harmed, given that the cycle of violence is escalating over time, given that it is difficult to stop the violence, why don't victims leave? Table 2 lists some of the common reasons that are given for not leaving. The fear of being killed or having one's children harmed are real fears.

TABLE 2. Why Don't They Leave
Fear of Being Killed
Fear for Safety of Children
No Financial Resources to Leave
Women's Shelters Will Not Take Teenage Children
Brainwashed into Believing that It Is His or Her Fault
Coerced to Stay
Believes Marriage Can Be Saved
Loves the Spouse
Stay Together for Good of Children
Too Embarrassed to Report It (Especially Males)
Shame

Batterers threaten to kill and do stalk and kill partners with chilling regularity. Other women do not have the financial resources and women's shelters will not take them in, if they have teenage children. Many victims have been brainwashed into thinking that they deserve this treatment (see the next section on torture) and others are coerced to stay by parents, neighbors, and the like. Some stay to save the marriages and some stay for the good of the children. Others, especially the males, are too embarrassed to report the domestic violence at all. Many male and female victims remain so out of shame. They were victims as children in their families of origin, perceive themselves to be damaged goods, and feel that they do not deserve better. None of them stays because he or she enjoys being punished, or becomes sexually aroused by being pushed around.

Torture. In truth, many are victims of torture just as if they had been tortured as prisoners of war in combat. Torture is the systematic, repetitive infliction of psychological fear to create disempowerment and disconnection. It is meant to instill terror and break the person's will. Batterers use the tools of any torturer: physical force, control of all information, threats of death or harm to self or others, unpredictable episodes of violence, capricious enforcement of petty rules, and destruction of the victim's sense of mastery by control of the victim's body and bodily functions (e.g., sleep, food, toilet, and exercise). The victim is especially kept away from all of the victim's friends, lest the victim hear some message discrepant with the assailant's message that the victim deserves his or her punishment. Over time the victim becomes brainwashed and believes the message. As we have seen in the sexual abuse of children and adults, physical abuse and battering can occur amongst any combination of relatives in the immediate or extended family. All of it is ugly and unacceptable.

Child Physical Abuse

Child abuse is equally grim and includes, in addition to sexual and physical abuse, neglect, abandonment, and murder. Forms of physical abuse may include physical battering, burning the child, tying up the child, overdosing the child on drugs, lacerating the child's legs with electric cord cuts, placing the child's buttocks on a stove's gas jet, and the like. There appears to be no end to what adults can think of to do to harm children.

The battering usually starts under age four, the mother is the most common assailant, and the hairbrush is the most common weapon. In these families, usually both parents were themselves victims of violence as children. They married young and had poor parenting skills. Often they have substance use disorders and are very socially isolated. In many cases the battered child was unwanted to begin with.

Signs of Abuse. It is instructive to note that, while the Society for the Prevention of Cruelty to Animals started at the turn of the 20th century, it was not until 1962 that Dr. C. Henry Kempe spelled out the child abuse syndrome (Kempe, Silverman, and Steele, 1962). Common signs of abuse include bruises; hidden marks or bruises not easily explained; unusual markings, such as those from cigarette burns; and a distended stomach, a sign of not being properly fed. Children at high risk for battering include congenitally malformed babies, premature babies, illegitimate babies, twins, and children of mothers with frequent pregnancies and excessive workloads.

Domestic Violence Murder

In some cases, the battering becomes no longer bearable or the burden of the child becomes overwhelming and murder may be the outcome. Following are two common examples.

In domestic violence situations between spouses, at some point the spouse may feel the need to stop the violence before he or she (or the children) would be killed. In these cases, the person waits until the assailant is distracted or asleep, and then implements a plan that the person has been considering for some time. In the absence of any imminent harm the spouse kills the partner. If the spouse is male, he will flee and likely commit suicide. If the spouse is female, she will call the police and turn herself in. In both cases, under current law, these spouses have committed murder because they had a premeditated plan and used excessive force in the absence of any imminent harm.

In the second example, many young teenage girls become pregnant to have a caring attachment. They wish for companionship but receive a complicated baby that has endless demands. The young woman feels burdened by the child rearing demands and realizes that she is less attractive to the males now that she has the baby. In circumstances like these, some mothers kill their children. Some may have postpartum depression, which complicates their reasoning but not all do.

The Intergenerational Transfer of Violence

If you were a child living in one of these violent dysfunctional families, you would want to get away as soon as you could. You would likely never want to see such violence again in your life nor in the lives of those you came to love at a later time. Yet the violence often continues from one generation to the next with a very high probability of its recurrence. Thoughtful research by C. S. Widom (1989) demonstrates that the likelihood of violence repeating itself in the next generation is 66 percent. How are we to understand this phenomenon?

Part of the explanation lies in knowing that domestic violence is one form of dysfunctional-family life and that dysfunctional families learn ways of behaving and strategies for coping that are not typical in more normal families.

Dysfunctional families have at least four rules that complicate the lives of their family members. The first rule is one of rigid control in dealing with the dysfunction. Families try to control and contain the dysfunction, whether it is battering, psychosis, substance use, gambling, philandering, and so forth. Every attempt is made to stop the behavior or at least keep it from spreading. This attempt at overcontrol results in rigid rules for containing the secret. The overcontrol is so extensive that, over time, other possible solutions to the problem are ruled out without even being considered.

The second family rule is one of secrecy. Family members are forbidden to discuss the family secret with anyone for fear of embarrassing the family in public. This emphasis on secrecy is closely linked to the third family rule, the rule of denial. Everyone in the family denies there is a problem, even to one another. Comments like "it's not that bad," "this happens in other families too," are examples of this form of denial and minimization. Members deny the problem as well as their own feelings of anger, anxiety, sadness, and shame about the problem.

The final rule is that of isolation. To keep the secret, to keep from being embarrassed, family members are encouraged to stay away from others, to keep their heads down, and go through life quietly and unobtrusively.

These rules result in family members who emphasize control at all costs, who do not know how they really feel, who have limited cognitive flexibility in problem-solving, and who are interpersonally skill deficient and socially isolated. These family members speak a foreign language compared to the rules that more normal families speak.

It is in this foreign-language tangle that the intergenerational transfer of violence may take root. The young people in domestic violence families want to grow up and move away from the violence, as we have noted. When they begin to date as teenagers, they are full of youthful idealism as was Joanne in the chapter vignette. They want change. They want a better life. However when they date, many dates feel uncomfortable because the dates are speaking the language of normal family rules for behavior. These dates think about how to solve problems, are not socially isolated, know how they feel, and actively solve problems. This feels like a foreign language to dysfunctional family members. The dysfunctional family teenagers do not realize that it is they who speak the foreign language, not everyone else. In the course of dating, by chance at some point they will meet another young adult from a dysfunctional family, as Joanne did, and it will feel "normal." Both will have the same set of dysfunctional family rules and they will understand each other and feel compatible.

Herein lies the crux of the problem. If they marry one another, each party will bring their set of dysfunctional family rules to the marriage and a new set of normal family problem-solving rules will not be learned. If verbal-conflict resolution skills are not learned, it should not be surprising that in the face of family conflicts the battery skills would reemerge. The intergenerational transfer of violence continues due to the absence of more adaptive problem-solving skills for life's inevitable problems.

Specific Safety Guidelines for Addressing Domestic Violence

In addition to the general safety intervention guidelines, we want to review some specific guidelines for domestic violence. As we have noted, this is one of the most dangerous situations that caregivers may encounter and we want to be sure that everyone is safe – patients and family members as well as caregivers.

Things to consider before arriving onsite. Think about the nature of the call, information in the admitting or call log, scene surveillance, and likely old brain stem prominence. It is likely that the stress of the domestic violence and its psychological impact on victims has resulted in fear and reduced higher cognitive function. Look for any early warning signs of loss of control in everyone in the room. Think of the various reasons anyone in the room might lose control. Has anyone been drinking? Are they hypervigilant, fearing the return of the assailant? Will children become angry if you remove the victim from the home because the children fear the return of the assailant? Are you removing the family's source of income? Is your presence in the neighborhood embarrassing the family? Finally, review the specific guidelines for approaching trauma victims that are outlined in the preceding chapter. It is quite likely that the victim(s) and some witnesses will be suffering from psychological trauma.

Onsite. Park beyond the house as we noted in the first chapter and account for everyone on the street. The assailant may be among them, if he or she has not been arrested. Approach the house and its door from its sides and listen for any signs of struggle. Are there loud voices? How many loud voices? Are any of the voices making specific threats?

As you enter, step to the sides of the door with your backs to the wall. If the fight is still in progress, separate the parties and move them in opposite directions. Separate them by tables and sofas and turn their backs to one another. Do not block your own exit route. Call the police for assistance. One team member keeps the assailant occupied as care is provided to the direct patient victim. Ask the assailant for a driver's license, health-insurance card, and so forth. Do not leave the assailant alone. If the assailant runs out, your team and the patient should leave also.

The Direct Victims. If circumstances permit (e.g., the assailant was earlier arrested and will not return during your visit), approach the victim patient as a victim of trauma. Use the guidelines for trauma victims from the previous chapter. Leave the victim space, explain who you are, ask permission to move closer to provide care, and explain each medical step. In this process, try to restore some sense of mastery in the victim by asking the victim to do something to help you with his or her own care.

Leaving the Home. **When you leave the home, assume that everyone in the home and in the street may be a potential assailant for any of the reasons noted above.** Search for early warning signs of loss of control and potential weapons and move quickly to the cover of your squad car, your ambulance, your motor vehicle, your emergency room, or your clinic.

We can see from the chapter vignette just how bad domestic violence situations can become. In many ways, Joanne is a prototypic illustration. Sexually and physically abused as a child, she became "a parentified child" with all of the problem-solving deficits, feeling states, and social isolation that young people experience growing up in a dysfunctional family. Her dysfunctional foreign language skills resulted in her overlooking the warning sign in William's past. The result was that the intergeneration transfer of violence continued in yet another family unit in spite of Joanne's efforts to prevent it.

The epigraph for this chapter notes that loneliness and the feeling of being unwanted are the most terrible poverty. When we respond to domestic violence situations, we may enhance the effectiveness of our own work if we keep in mind that caring family attachments have been shattered and that family feelings are raw. Extra kindness and outreach by those of us providing care will make our own work easier but may also result in the patient or client trusting the care system so that, in time, he or she is able to extricate herself or himself from the dysfunction of domestic violence. Table 3 presents a bullet summary of our general and specific safety guidelines to this point.

TABLE 3. Safety Guidelines

- *Think Medical and Psychiatric Illness*
- *Think Call Log*
- *Think Scene Surveillance*
- *Think Old Brain Stem*
- *Think Early Warning Signs*
- *Think Theories of Violence*
- *Think Psychological Trauma*
- *Think Domestic Violence*

The next chapter reviews psychiatric emergencies, especially the puzzle of psychosis and why persons with psychotic illnesses often exhibit strange behaviors. Since many of these psychotic individuals do not realize that they have psychosis, when it first begins, many self-medicate their symptoms with drugs or alcohol just as many victims of trauma also do. The next chapter, therefore, will also include a short review of the problem of substance use and abuse.

FIVE

Psychiatric Emergencies/ Substance Use

My peace is gone. My heart is heavy.

—Johann Wolfgang von Goethe

"What does she think this is, anyway? A hotel?" asked Naomi Fuller of no one in particular. Naomi was the residential house manager of a neighborhood home for eight persons with serious mental illness. Managing such a home was complex enough and now she had one of the residents staying out all night every night.

Maria, the resident in question, had a long history of being physically abusive toward others, making frightening verbal threats to others, and generally being hostile to everyone that she met. Maria had come to the residence just two months ago. She appeared to have adjusted well until the third month. Then it all began. Each late afternoon she would take her evening meal from the kitchen and place it in a brown paper bag. Abrupt with others even in the best of times, she would then loudly announce that she was going out, regardless of what others thought. She took the city bus downtown and did not return until seven o'clock the next morning. She would sleep all day, do her house chores, pack another dinner, and then leave again for the city.

Naomi was both angry and sick with worry about Maria. After all, Maria had a serious mental illness and a long history of violence. What was she doing all night? Drugs? Gambling? Prostitution?

One cool, October evening, Naomi followed Maria at a distance. Maria got off the city bus and went to a city park that was known to house the homeless at night, when the important-seeming people had abandoned the park for the suburbs. Naomi watched as Maria sat down beside a man wrapped in a blanket and fed him her dinner.

The next morning Naomi was at the residence to meet Maria, when she returned. "What is this all about, Maria?" asked Naomi quietly. "It's none of your damn business, is it?" was Maria's curt reply. Then Maria's voice softened. "He's my boyfriend. He has no money for food, so I feed him. He has no place to live, so I sit with him so that he doesn't have to be alone in the darkness of the night."

Naomi wept uncontrollably.

This chapter might have begun with some of the more common behavioral emergencies such as Maria's being assaultive or Richard's behavioral disorganization in the police standoff noted in chapter 2. However, I choose to focus on her kindness and compassion for others, even in the face of her own difficulties, so that we may begin to address the issue of stigma as well as her psychiatric illness.

In psychiatric emergencies that involve psychosis, persons with these illnesses have a brain-based, genetic illness that results in unusual, strange, and, at times, violent frightening behaviors. These behaviors include hearing voices that are not there; seeing events that are not there; having false, often paranoid beliefs about oneself or others; disrobing in public; speaking in sentences that others cannot understand; having intense feelings of anger or depression; having strong body odor; and, at times, becoming assaultive. These patients do not want to behave in this fashion but without proper medications they have no volitional capacity to control what is happening to them. All of these unusual behaviors are tedious, and some are truly frightening, such as when the voices are telling you to kill a family member before that family member destroys you. On average, these patients die ten years earlier than the average person. Some lives are shortened by one's own hand; some, from lifestyle issues; some, from medical diseases not attended to because of psychotic states untreated over several years.

Not only are these behaviors distressing to persons with psychotic illnesses, they are distressing to average citizens who do not understand these unusual behaviors as symptoms of medical illnesses that need to be and can be treated. Citizens feel ill-at-ease, frightened, and confused by these behaviors. To gain some illusion of control of the situation, citizens sometimes ridicule and stigmatize these ill patients. *Stigma* comes from the Latin word for "mark," a mark of shame or discredit. To gain control of their own anxiety about these unusual behaviors, citizens orally abuse, make fun of, ridicule, threaten, and disparage these patients to their face and in front of others. Such public mockery is a very painful, additional burden. This stigmatizing is found in all levels of society, including health care.

Four decades of treating persons with serious mental illness has taught many of us at least two important lessons. The first is that these patients are people first. They have the same hopes, aspirations, excitements, and heartaches that the rest of us do, even if their goals are complicated by a genetically inherited brain disability.

The second lesson is that of the extraordinary goodness and kindness that they offer to one another, such as that shown by Maria. Their illnesses have complicated life's goals but they have fallen in love and cared for one another, they have married and raised children; they have helped one another when their psychiatric illnesses have flared up; they have buried their parents and siblings; they have nursed loved ones through death; and they have demonstrated extreme grace under pressure in the face of ignorant, stigmatizing, derogation by others.

When health-care providers respond to psychiatric behavioral emergencies, we want to focus on fully understanding which psychiatric illness is being suggested by the unusual behaviors before us and we want to be sure to educate any citizen on the street or any person in our waiting rooms to avoid ignorant statements, so that our patient does not have to endure being stigmatized, even as we go about providing care.

This chapter examines psychiatric behavioral emergencies and includes the main types, common problematic behaviors, the necessary medications for successful treatment, and the serious side effects of these medications. As noted, since many of these patients self-medicate their symptoms with substances, we shall examine briefly the main drugs of abuse and their withdrawal symptoms. Finally, suicide among the seriously mentally ill is much higher than in the general population and we shall close with an overview of this important risk factor to be monitored. All psychiatric and substance use syndromes discussed in this chapter may be examined in greater detail in the diagnostic manual of the American Psychiatric Association (1994).

The General Nature of Psychiatric Emergencies

The numbers and types of psychiatric disorders are many and varied. All of them cause psychological distress in some way and most can be successfully treated. Usually, these illnesses do not result

FIGURE 1. Continuum of Psychiatric Disorders

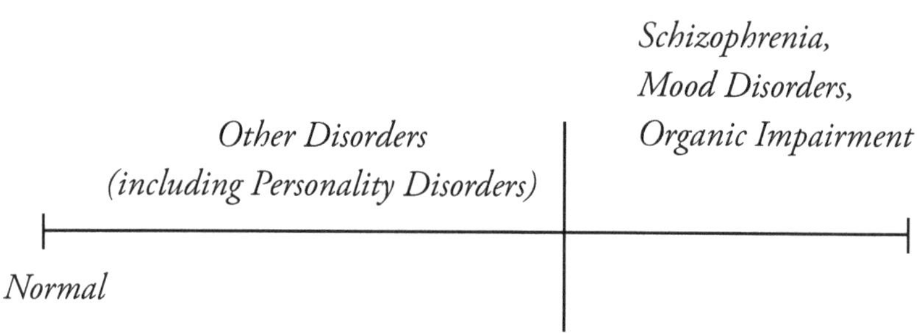

in behavioral emergencies. Figure 1 presents a simplified way to remember the psychiatric conditions that may result in behavioral emergencies.

Here is a continuum of increasing severity from normal to other disorders (including personality disorders) to schizophrenia, mood disorders, and organic impairment. These are demarcated by a solid line that cuts through the continuum line. This line is meant to indicate the genetic-based illnesses that manifest themselves under severe life-stress (schizophrenia, mood disorders) or permanent injury to the brain (organic impairment). We will include an overview of each of these three very serious conditions as well as a short section on the main personality disorders that may be involved in some additional types of behavioral emergencies.

The Nature of Serious Mental Illnesses

Schizophrenia. Schizophrenia is a genetic illness that manifests itself primarily in disturbances in cognition. Communicating is illogical and incoherent sentences and paragraphs may be one sign of this problem. Another common sign is the altered sense perceptions called hallucinations. Persons with schizophrenia may see things that are not there, hear things that are not there, or smell things that are not there. In addition, they may also have false beliefs about themselves or others. These are called *delusions* and are often paranoid or persecutory in nature. At other times, the patient may become grandiose and perceive him or herself as an important person. Sometimes these patients engage in grossly disorganized, bizarre behaviors. Many express little emotion, limited motivation, and limited interest in socializing with others.

Mood Disorders. Mood disorders manifest themselves in extreme and overwhelming feeling states. Some mood disorders may be due to substance abuse or medical conditions, but here our focus is on those that appear to be genetic. These may include *major depressive disorders* with marked depressed mood, diminished interest in almost all activities, significant weight loss, insomnia, psychomotor agitation or retardation, fatigue, feelings of worthlessness, and recurrent thoughts of death or suicide. Depressive disorders may occur only once or may recur, often in some temporal pattern, such as in two-year cycles.

Bipolar Disorder may include manic episodes. Patients with mania have a persistently elevated or irritable mood that lasts at least one week. They may have inflated self-esteem or feelings of grandiosity, be more talkative then usual, have racing thoughts, and be easily distractible. They may also have excessive involvement in pleasurable activities that may have painful consequences, such as sexual indiscretions or buying sprees. Persons with bipolar mood disorders may have both the manic and depressed components of this disease. In addition, some individuals have both a schizophrenic and a mood disorder and this is known as schizoaffective disorder.

Organic Impairment. Organic impairment refers to destruction of tissue in the brain, especially in the cortex or the limbic system. Reasoning, memory, orientation, accurate sense perception, and coordinated motor behavior may all be disrupted. The site of the injury often results in the corresponding brain deficit. We saw some common examples in table 2 in chapter 1, in such medical conditions as Alzheimer's disease, traumatic brain injury, multi-infarct dementia, and stroke.

The gross disorganization and impairment in schizophrenia, mood disorders, and organic impairment often result in behavioral emergency situations with the accompanying possibility of violence.

Personality Disorders. As we mentioned in passing in chapter 2, personality disorders are ingrained patterns of behavior and coping that are maladaptive either to the patient or to those with whom the patient is interacting. They would be grouped under "Other Disorders" in figure 1 and do not have clear genetic bases. Those that may be involved in behavioral emergency calls include antisocial, borderline, narcissistic and paranoid disorders.

Antisocial persons fail to conform to society norms; are deceitful; impulsive; irresponsible; have little concern for people and property; and may be aggressive, as indicated by repeated fights and assaults.

Persons with borderline personality disorder go to great lengths to avoid real or imagined abandonment, have unstable interpersonal relations that idolize or devalue the other, have an unstable sense of self, recurring impulsive behaviors, recurring suicidal behavior, and marked periods of irritable and intense anger that may result in assaultiveness.

Narcissistic individuals have an enhanced sense of self-importance, are preoccupied with success and power, are entitled, lack empathy, and exploit others.

The paranoid personality disordered person is suspicious of others; is preoccupied with the trustworthiness of others; is reluctant to socialize with others in basic, common social interactions; bears grudges; and may react angrily to counteract perceived injustices.

Since each of these personality disorders may include assaultiveness as one of their components, it is clear why they are included in possible behavioral emergencies.

The Biology of the Serious Mental Illnesses

The complex biochemistry of these various medical conditions is beyond the scope of this book. However, a review of the basic structures in the brain (figure 5, chapter 1) and the synaptic-gap nerve transmission system (figure 1, chapter 3) will enable us to understand a basic sense of what causes these illnesses.

Schizophrenia. In truth, the etiology of schizophrenia remains unknown at this time. Several researchers are studying various brain structures and different types of neurotransmitters. One widely research theory is the dopamine hypothesis, which hypothesizes that there is too much of a neurotransmitter called dopamine in the synaptic gaps in the limbic system and too little dopamine in the synaptic gaps in the prefrontal cortex. Theoretically, dopamine is thought to interfere with the normal transmission of messages in the brain and to result in many of the cognitive abnormalities that we have noted.

Mood Disorders. There is more widespread consensus on the etiology of manic and depressive states and that they likely occur in the limbic system. Mania appears to result from the absence of ordinary common table salt in the synaptic gaps. However, giving sodium chloride (ordinary table salt) to persons with mania does not appear to result in its being absorbed into the person's synaptic gaps and salt substitutes must be employed. Depressive states appear to manifest themselves when serotonin is depleted and may lead to suicidal behaviors, if serotonin is severely depleted.

Organic impairments result from damage to brain tissue and the brain structures. Cerebral vascular accidents, encephalitis, infections, tumors, lead poisoning, and various types of head injuries are some of the possible precipitants to organic brain impairment. As we noted earlier, there is no clear biological basis at this time for the personality disorders.

Common Psychiatric Medications in Serious Mental Illnesses

There are many varieties of psychiatric medications. Table 1 (adapted from the Massachusetts Department of Mental Health *Medication Information Manual* [2007]) lists some of the more common agents by both generic and trade names. Antipsychotic medications are used for treating schizophrenia and consist of traditional medications, as well as some more recent advances known as atypicals. Mood stabilizers are utilized to reduce manic states and the three types of antidepressant medications are used to lessen depressive states. Often patients may be able to tell you which medications have been prescribed for them or they may have a vial of medicine on their person. The information in table 1 may prove to be valuable in helping you ascertain the person's psychiatric illness.

Side Effects

Many of these agents have side effects. Low-level side effects include drowsiness, dizziness, constipation, dry mouth, sleep disturbance, weight gain, diarrhea, and thermal dysregulation. These side effects are nettlesome but are tolerable. Some side effects, however, may

TABLE 1. Common Psychiatric Medications (Generic and Trade Names)

Antipsychotic Medications

Traditional Agents

Generic	Trade
Chlorpromazine	Thorazine
Fluphenazine	Prolixin
Haloperidol	Haldol
Perphenazine	Trilafon
Trifluoperazine	Stelazine
Thioridazine	Mellaril

Newer Agents

Generic	Trade
Clozapine	Clozaril
Olanzapine	Zyprexa
Quetiapine	Seroquel
Risperidone	Risperidal

Mood Stabilizers

Generic	Trade
Carbamazepine	Tegretol
Divalproex Sodium	Depakote
Gabapentin	Neurontin
Lamotigine	Lamictal
Lithium Carbonate	Lithofid
Topirimate	Topamax
Valproic Acid	Depakene

Antidepressant Medications

Monoamine Oxidase Inhibitors (MAOIs)

Generic	Trade
Phenelzine	Nardil
Tranylcypromine	Parnate

Selective Serotonin Re-Uptake Inhibitors (SSRIs)

Generic	Trade
Citaloprom	Celexa
Fluoxetine	Prozac
Paroxitine	Paxil
Sertraline	Zoloft

Tricyclic Antidepressants (TCAP)

Generic	Trade
Amitriptyline	Elavil
Doxepin	Sinequan
Imiprimine	Trofranil

Other Psychoactive Medications

Anticholinergies

Generic	Trade
Benztropine	Cogentin
Trihexphenidyl	Artane

Beta Blockers

Generic	Trade
Metoprolol	Lopressor
Propranolol	Inderal

TABLE 2. Serious Medication Side Effects

Agrangular Cytosis
Cardiovascular Disease
Cataracts
Diabetes
Dysphagia
Extrapyramidal Side Effects
  Akathesia
  Akinesia
  Dystonic Reaction
  Dyskinesia/Tardiff Dyskinesia
  Neuroleptic Malignant Syndrome
Polydypsia
Rotted Teeth

result in serious bodily disruptions, and some, even in death. Table 2 presents some of the more common, serious side effects.

Agrangular cytosis is a lowering of a person's white blood-cell count in response to clozapine. It impairs the person's immune system and places the person at risk for infection. It can be fatal. Cardiovascular medical issues may arise from several different types of medications, such as thioridazine and chlorpromazine, and may manifest themselves in several different types of cardiovascular illness. Cataracts may form in some patients who are taking quetiapine. Diabetes may arise in patients prescribed the new atypicals, such as clozapine and olanzapine. Dysphagia is the inability to swallow correctly and smoothly and may result in choking and gagging. Many of these agents lead to dysphagia over time. Polydypsia is severe thirst and, again, is associated with the use of many antipsychotic medicines over time. Similarly, rotted teeth may emerge from the use of lithium salts also over a protracted period of time.

Many of the antipsychotic medications lead to a dysregulation of dopamine and choline in the basal ganglia in the old brain stem. These deregulations result in extrapyramidal side effects and result in a variety of disruptions in motor behaviors. Akathesia is restless behavior and the inability to sit still. Akinesia is the lack of movement. Dystonic reactions result in muscle spasms. Dyskinesia results in repetitive motor movements, such as twitches or eye blinking. A serious type of dyskinesia is tardiff dyskinesia in which the patient has involuntary moments of the mouth, jaw, and tongue.

Of the dyskinesias, neuroleptic malignant syndrome is the most serious of the extrapyramidal side effects. Like agrangular cytosis, neuroleptic malignant syndrome may result in death. The syndrome is characterized by fever, muscle stiffness, changes in blood pressure and heart rate, and thermal desregulation in the hypothalamus that results in a release of chemicals that destroy the brain and liver tissue. Again, antipsychotic medications may result in this syndrome.

This brief overview illustrates the power of these agents and the daily decisions that must be made by patients with these serious mental illness. They strive to find the balance between clear cognition and normal feeling states and at the same time avoid the medication side effects that can greatly impair health. These are difficult illnesses to bear.

Given the unpleasant side effects of these medications, some patients stop taking them. This is especially true of young adults who do not want to accept that they have a chronic illness in the first place. The potency of many of these medications is reduced substantially after a period of thirty days. At that point, medication noncompliance states may appear as acute disorganized states of schizophrenia and mood disorders. The noncompliant patient may also be self-medicating with drugs or alcohol and showing signs of increased agitation with the potential for assaultiveness, increased suicidality, increased disorganized thinking, and depressed or euphoric mood states. Care-providers want to assess patients involved in behavioral emergencies for medication noncompliance and substance use. Ask patients when they took their last dose of prescribed medication and how much of it they took. Ask if they have been using drugs.

Substance Use Disorders

Individuals use alcohol and other forms of drugs to modify feeling states of anger, anxiety, depression, boredom, and the like. They are self-medicating dysphoric states with the goal of increasing more pleasant feeling states, such as calmness, joy, peace, and pleasurable excitement, to name a few. This self-medication process usually becomes more frequent and worse over time and may result in both psychological and physical addictions. Medicine and the behavioral sciences refer to these negative end states as substance use disorders. The field has learned over time that negative physical and psychological health consequences may occur at any point in the self-medication process. Hence the current terminology of substance use as opposed to substance abuse, which often implies advanced physical addiction.

There are a great many prescripted medications and unprescripted street drugs in our society. Four common ones that are often present during behavioral emergencies are alcohol, crack/

TABLE 3. Drug Abuse: Possible Warning Signs

Bodily States	Poor Motor Coordination, Slurred Speech, Shallow Breathing, Glazed Eyes, Dilated Pupils Decreased Alertness, Drowsiness Loss of Appetite, Disturbed Sleep, Loss of Libido
Feeling States	Depression, Hostility, Irritability, Elation
Behaviors	Appears Intoxicated, Dark Glasses, Drug Paraphernalia, Long Sleeves

cocaine, methamphetamine, and opioids. Table 3 lists some of the more common warning signs.

Alcohol. Alcohol seeps into the synaptic gaps of the nervous system and results in disrupted functioning that includes ataxias, slurred speech, anesthetized memory (blackouts), impaired attention and judgment, and stupor or coma. Withdrawal symptoms may include autonomic hyperactivity (sweating, increased pulse > 100), insomnia, nausea or vomiting, transient hallucinations, psychomotor agitation, and tonic-clonic (grand mal) seizures.

Crack/Cocaine. These drugs stimulate the dopamine neurotransmitter system until the dopamine is depleted. Disrupted functioning may include dilated pupils, tachycardia or bradycardia, blood pressure alterations, perspiration or chills, nausea or vomiting, weight loss, psychomotor agitation or retardation, muscular weaknesses, cardiac arrhythmias, confusion, seizure, or coma, among others. Withdrawal symptoms include fatigue, unpleasant dreams, insomnia or hypersomnia, psychomotor retardation or agitation, and increased appetite.

Methamphetamine. Similar to cocaine, methamphetamines also deplete the dopamine neurotransmitter system. Common signs of use include tachycardia or bradycardia, dilated pupils, blood pressure alterations, perspiration or chills, nausea or vomiting, psychomotor agitation or retardation, confusion, seizures, dyskinesias, dystonias, and coma. Withdrawal symptoms may include fatigue, unpleasant dreams, insomnia or hypersomnia, increased appetite, and psychomotor retardation or agitation.

Opioids. Opioids appear to stimulate subcortical receptors in the central nervous system and in the gastrointestinal system. Signs of use include initial euphoria followed by apathy or dysphoria; psychomotor agitation or retardation; impaired judgment; pupil constriction; and drowsiness, coma, or slurred speech. Opiate withdrawal includes dysphoric mood, nausea or vomiting, muscle aches, pupil dilate, diarrhea, fever, and insomnia.

Clearly, the use and abuse of alcohol and drugs carries important and serious health risks in their use and in their withdrawal states. Compounding these matters further is that many substance users are also heavy users of caffeine and nicotine, drugs that make negative health consequences even more likely. Cortical disinhibition from these substances increases the risk of violent behaviors.

Suicide

Living with the serious mental illnesses of schizophrenia and mood disorders, and/or with their powerful medications and negative side effects is a burden. Self-medicating these illnesses with drugs, alcohol, caffeine, and nicotine brings additional serious health risks. Add to this the social isolation experienced by many of these patients, and the ongoing stigma by others, and even the most sturdy soul may become overwhelmed. Suicide may emerge as a path in many cases, far more than would be the case in the normal population. The depression, the desperation, the lack of any perceived hope leads some to take their own lives as we noted in chapter 3.

Medicine and behavioral science have documented some of the most common risk factors for health-care providers to consider in evaluating suicide potential during behavioral emergencies. For persons with schizophrenia, these include current life-stress, the severity of the psychiatric symptoms, delusions (especially those of persecution or control, noncompliance with medications, extrapyramidal symptoms, and past or present suicidal behavior. For persons with mood disorders, a co-occurring substance use disorder, a previous suicide attempt, a family history of suicide, and access to lethal weapons are important risk factors. Social supports (caring attachments), having children, having religious beliefs, and having a meaningful purpose in life are buffers that mitigate the risk factors in both illnesses.

Caregivers may want to ask the four following questions of persons considered at risk for suicide:

1. "Do you want to hurt yourself? Yes? No?" If the person says "yes," do not leave the person alone and take the person to an emergency room. If the person says "no," ask the second question.

2. "If you did want to hurt yourself, how would you do it?" Here you are listening for the person's plan. In general, the more detailed the plan, the more likely the person might be to act on it. Next ask the third question.
3. "What keeps you alive?" Here you are listening for the buffering factors that would dissuade the person from self-harm.
4. Finally, ask the last question. "Has it been helpful to discuss this?" If the person says that speaking has been helpful and the suicidal stress has been lessened, the risk may now be less but should be evaluated in light of the information from the other three questions. If the person is at high risk based on his or her answers to these questions and has found no relief in speaking about these matters, do not leave the person alone and take the person to the nearest emergency room for further evaluation and treatment.

Should you encounter a behavioral emergency in which the patient or client is threatening homicide, take cover and call for immediate police assistance. If it is possible from a position of safety, try to engage the homicidal person in conversation. Try to ascertain the homicidal person's perceived grievance and the intended victim to have this information for the police. If you can, keep the homicidal person talking, until the police arrive. If the assailant flees, work with the police to alert the intended victim and others that may be bystanders in the area.

Specific Safety Guidelines for Addressing Psychiatric Emergencies/Substance Use

As was the case in dealing with psychological trauma and domestic violence, we begin with the general safety guidelines. To the extent that such information is known, what is the nature of the behavioral emergency illness that has generated the call for assistance? Does the admitting chart or call log have any relevant information, including previous requests for this same patient or client? Onsite, a thorough scene analysis is in order and an awareness that the patient may be primarily old brain-stem dominant should be considered. The patient should also be monitored for any of the early warning signs of loss of control. Finally, we want to be considering any possible theories of violence that might explain the current potential for violence, so that we can diffuse it before it occurs. For example, in the case of a paranoid patient, what immediate steps might be taken to reduce the patient's fear of being harmed?

If there is no immediate medical crisis or violent behavior in the psychiatric or substance use emergency, form as best one can an alliance with the patient. Emphasize that together you can solve the problem without violence. When we caregivers arrive onsite, we need to remember that patients may see us as representing either jail or long-term hospitalization and they will not necessarily be eager to work with us. Forming an alliance may result in the patient being more cooperative.

Until proven otherwise, assume that the patient or client is a victim of psychological trauma. Follow the guidelines for assisting trauma victims. Keep a distance. Respect shattered trauma boundaries. Speak in clear, simple, direct questions and statements. Restore the person's sense of mastery quickly in whatever way presents itself.

Since this is a psychiatric and/or substance use disorder behavioral emergency, health-care providers will want to add the following specific guidelines. Assess for signs of schizophrenia, mood disorders, and/or organic impairment. Assess for the presence of any medications or information about current medications. Monitor for signs of medication noncompliance or any of the serious medication side effects, especially neuroleptic malignant syndrome. As you are evaluating these issues, assess also for the presence of substance use and any withdrawal symptoms, if indicated. Finally, assess for the presence of suicidal thoughts and behaviors, especially in those individuals who have a thorough and potentially workable plan to harm oneself. Many assaults and injuries occur during psychiatric behavioral emergencies with the imposition of restraints. We shall examine alternatives to restraints in chapter 7.

As a general rule, if it is safe to do so, transport the patient to the ER without the use of restraints.

Most police jurisdictions have two common law rules that permit them to take responsibility for a person with a psychiatric emergency. Police have the power and authority to take responsibility for mental illness in the community and *parens patrie* obligations to protect individuals with disabilities.

One tragic and painful reality of schizophrenia and mood disorders is that these illnesses frequently flare up. Sometimes the flare up is due to medication noncompliance but more frequently it is a function of the illnesses themselves and/or extreme life-stress. By middle-age, a person with one of these illnesses may have had between ten and thirty hospital admissions, which represents several years of being institutionalized in public and private hospitals.

When we met Maria at the beginning of this chapter, she was somewhat irritable at times but was basically a higher-functioning middle-aged adult who was concerned with the needs of others. Had we been called during one of her psychiatric flare-ups, what might we have encountered? Maria has schizoaffective disorder, so we would likely have had disordered logic, paranoid delusions, depression, and true hostility. If this state of disorganization had been present for a few days, Maria would also likely have started using alcohol to self-medicate her psychiatric distress. As we are called to assist, she might be manifesting symptoms of alcohol use and she may well be suicidal, as she is depressed and this would be her twenty-seventh admission. As we treat the various components of this clinical picture, it may be helpful to bear in mind that this person is the same soul that fed the hungry and that she can be returned to that same high level of functioning with adequate treatment. This treatment very much includes our own efforts during the behavioral emergency, treatments that will provide high quality care in the absence of stigma. Patients are grateful for such care and concern.

Table 4 is a chapter summary of the general and specific safety guidelines to address the material that we have covered thus far.

TABLE 4. Safety Guidelines

- *Think Medical and Psychiatric Illness*
- *Think Call Log*
- *Think Scene Surveillance*
- *Think Old Brain Stem*
- *Think Early Warning Signs*
- *Think Theories of Violence*
- *Think Psychological Trauma*
- *Think Domestic Violence*
- *Think Psychiatric Emergency/Substance Use/ Suicide*

We now turn to the last of the commonly encountered behavioral emergencies that we are called to respond to: that of youth violence and other forms of criminal activity. Violence among young people is a serious national public-health issue. We need to recognize its early warning signs so that we can prevent its cruption in school shootings, gang warfare, and the like.

SIX

Youth Violence/Crime

The heart has reason that reason knows not of.

—Blaise Pascal

Jennifer hadn't wanted to get up this morning. It was the anniversary date and she was saddened by the thought of it. Funny, how you didn't forget some calls. Already it had been a year since Kurt and she in their advance life support unit had been dispatched to the corner of Granger and Franklin Avenues. The call had been one of the most publicized youth shootings in the city the year before. A fifteen-year-old boy, a good boy, was gunned down on Granger Avenue on his way to the YMCA to play basketball after school. Jennifer and Kurt worked feverishly with all of their paramedic skills to strengthen a failing pulse. Her hand was shaking as she wrote his name in the log book, Jerome Dalia, and she fought back tears as they raced to the nearest emergency room. Dead on arrival. It was depressing then. It was depressing today.

It was also depressing this morning in the Dalia household on Wolcott Road. Mrs. Dalia thought that there was nothing of her heart left to break. Yet here on the anniversary date of her son's death, the vice-like grip of pain from grief crushed her chest. Jerome's sister, Charlene, was determined to visit the small, makeshift memorial to her brother that had sprung up in the neighborhood in her brother's memory – a few dead flowers, a broken hockey stick, some curbside dust. She wanted to honor his memory on this first anniversary.

"Unit 6, immediate dispatch to Granger and Franklin Avenues." Kurt and Jennifer looked at each other in total disbelief, as the dispatch was repeated. Onsite where the body of Jerome had lain the year before was the body of a nineteen-year-old female, similarly an innocent victim of a gang drive-by shooting. When Jennifer was told the identity of the victim, her hand shook so violently that a nearby police officer had to write the patient's name in her logbook, Charlene Dalia. In the back of the truck, Jennifer cried openly as she and Kurt again raced in the heart of darkness to an emergency room for a miracle that no emergency room would be able to provide.

Youth violence is hardly new or a phenomenon. From clay tablets in ancient Mesopotamia to the Middle Ages, to our own day, societal observers have written about turbulent, rebellious, and violent youth (Baker and Rubel; 1980, Volokch and Snell, 1998). What is new is the extent and lethality of this violence in today's scientifically advanced age.

Although there is adult organized crime and some hardened, adult career criminals, a large percentage of a society's violence and crime is usually committed in any generation by those in the age range of fifteen-to-twenty-four years. Although many factors affect the crime rate, the size of this age cohort is one important contributing factor. Other things being equal, the larger this cohort is, the more likely will be the presence of crime and violence in that society.

Recent years have seen a continuing increase in youth violence in the United States, Europe, and the Middle East, countries in which such information is kept. These youths are committing the major felonies of homicides, rapes, (armed) robberies, and assaults. The lethality of these crimes has increased as guns have replaced fistfights for the resolution of conflict. Some citizens in the United States think of youth violence as high-school students shooting up their schools, teachers, and classmates. These shootings occur primarily in rural settings. Other citizens consider youth violence to be the mayhem that occurs in poverty-stricken, drug-inflated urban neighborhoods, where life on the street is one of constant survival in the jungle. Most all citizens are startled when this rural and urban jungle violence is disrupted by youth in affluent suburbs. Each viewpoint is correct.

What are the causes of this continuing presence of youth violence? In addition to the theories of violence, is there any way to identify those youth inclined to follow violent pathways? Why are both poverty and affluence involved in youth violence? Is there any way to reach these children before violence erupts? What happens to youth who witness the violence committed by other youths? Do these young witnesses remain overwhelmed? Do they ever recover? Do they themselves go on to become violent? And what is the role of professional health-care providers, when asked to assist assailant victims, innocent victims, and victim witnesses? Will the well-intended professional also be attacked in the performance of duties?

In this chapter, we shall pursue initial answers to these questions, as we examine the complex factors that need to be considered in these assessments. As in the three preceding chapters, we will close with specific safety guidelines for caregivers so that we may both survive and provide care in this jungle. Let us review what medicine and behavioral science can tell us about these youthful assailants.

The Youthful Offender

Since the youth of each generation commit a disproportional amount of society's crime and violence, a considerable amount of research in medicine and behavioral science has been directed over the decades toward enhancing our understanding of why many young people are so prone to violence.

Let us begin with what the theories of violence can teach us about troubled youth. First, it is clear that the cultural context of *anomie,* as identified by Émile Durkheim, affects all of today's young people, including those who become violent. We live in an age of rapid social change, as we have seen, and this change is coupled with the newly emerging cultural values of oneself first, material goods, and instant gratification. This has resulted in an anomic society with no clear rules for socially acceptable behavior with the resultant emergence of disrespect for others as well as a general loss of community cohesiveness. Youth involved in crime in today's age have less guidance, less oversight, and fewer rules from adults about what constitutes acceptable social behavior.

There are a number of biological factors that have been reported in youthful offenders. These include hyperreactivity to the environment, abnormal electroencephalograph (EEG) readings, attention deficit hyperactivity disorder, untreated posttraumatic stress disorder, a variety of substance use disorders, and possibly genetic/social dysfunction factors. Similar research on the sociological factors associated with violence in youth have noted the prominence of dysfunctional families, where empathic skills may not be taught, the role of both poverty and affluence, poor schooling and truancy, discrimination, substance use disorders, and readily obtainable weapons.

Research in the psychological factors of mastery and motivational values suggest mixed findings in terms of mastery. In general, youthful assailants are deficient in personal care and interpersonal skills. However, a number of them have street smarts and rely on this communication system for daily living. With regard to academic skills, many are school dropouts and are unable to obtain work in the postindustrial state. In their teenage years they have already become members of the permanent underclass. However, others, while lacking formal schooling, are innately bright and are particularly good in criminal entrepreneurial businesses like running a drugs cartel at a profit. In terms of the other psychological dimension of values and motivation for behavior, many espouse the antisocial values that we noted in chapter 2.

Although these research findings on the theories of violence present a broad array of possible delinquent youth characteristics, an important paradox remains. There are many youth who have many of these same characteristics in their lives and yet never became violent. They remain law-abiding young adults. Faced with this paradox, a criminologist, Dr. Marvin Wolfgang, and his research colleagues adopted a new research approach (Wolfgang, Figlio, and Sellin, 1972). Instead of studying youthful offenders after the fact, they would study the development of delinquency as it emerged after birth, a prospective study to see how neonates go bad.

Dr. Wolfgang and his colleagues recorded the births of all males in the city of Philadelphia in 1945. The births included 9,945 male babies who were then followed by the research team unit they reached their eighteenth birthdays. The research team recorded any encounters that these children had with the police. Two-thirds of the subjects had no involvement with the police in any way. Of the remaining thirty-five percent, half had committed one delinquent or criminal act and had no further involvement. Two-thirds of the other half had two or more encounters before their eighteenth birthdays. However, 627 were arrested five or more times. This small group of core offenders, as they have become known, committed a disproportionately large percentage of all serious crimes in the city. This eighteen-year study was repeated again including both males and females and children of all races (Tracy, Wolfgang, and Figlio, 1990). The findings were the same. A small group of core offenders were committing an unacceptably high percentage of the city's serious crimes. So robust was this finding, that policing agencies throughout the county now focus their crime prevention efforts in identifying and imprisoning these core youthful offenders in any given jurisdiction. However, Dr. Wolfgang and his colleagues did not study what made these core offenders engage in criminal behavior.

The Continuum of Youth Warning Signs

As researchers focused on the various theories associated with youth violence, and as Wolfgang's colleagues focused on two cohorts over time, my own research focused on a review on the longitudinal studies of juvenile delinquents that have been undertaken since the 1890s to see if potential youth assailants could be more fully understood. There have been ten major such studies and they encompass the characteristics of 10,800 delinquent youths (Flannery, 2000).

When youth violence occurs, neighbors ask how could this happen? The child and his or her family were good people. Why were there no warning signs? These ten studies reveal that in fact there are warning signs. Sometimes there are many warning signs and often they have been there for years. Even more startling is the fact that the warning signs have been the same for this century of studies. Even though the world we live in has been plagued by wars and has advanced through periods of great technological change, the signs of troubled children prone to violence have remained the same over the years.

As I reviewed these warning signs, it appeared to me that they could be arranged on a continuum of severity from Early Warning Signs through Serious Warning Signs to Urgent Warning Signs. Table 1 presents an outline of the warning signs and their various components. The continuum on the left reflects the increasing severity as one proceeds down the column. What appears of importance in understanding and preventing youth violence is that actual violence itself emerges during the Urgent Warning Signs. This suggests

TABLE 1. The Continuum of Warning Signs

Early Warning Signs	Disruptions in Attachments Disruptions in Mastery Disruptions in Meaningful Purpose
Serious Warning Signs	Depression/Suicide Substance use disorder Posttraumatic Stress Disorder
Urgent Warning Signs	Conduct Disorder

that there are many warning signs present much earlier on. Since this is a continuum of progression toward violence, there may be ways over the course of many years to identify those children at risk for violence and to intervene before such violence actually occurs.

Preliminary Considerations

Since no one can predict violence with one-hundred-percent accuracy, this continuum of warning signs does not predict which specific children will go on to become violent. Rather, it is better to consider the warning signs as probabilities of potential violence: the more the warning signs, the greater the likelihood of crime or violence. It is important to remember that all of these warning signs reflect an underlying issue that is hurtful to the child. Since the warning signs are there for some time before violence may erupt, adults who train themselves to identify the warning signs have a much greater opportunity to help the troubled child early on. Finally, it is helpful to remember that the more severe the signs become, the more difficult and lengthy will be the treatments for remediation. Helping a child with the early warning sign reduces the possibility for violence, shortens the period of suffering for the child, increases the probability of successful resolution, and is more cost-effective and efficient in terms of treatment interventions.

The Early Warning Signs

Noted earlier is the importance of caring attachments, reasonable mastery, and a meaningful sense of purpose as contributing to a person's good physical and mental health. All of these domains of good health may be disrupted amid the early warning signs.

Caring Attachments. Caring attachments to others can be disrupted in any of several ways. First are the physical disruptions of family caring attachments. In this grouping, the intact family is actually broken and dissolved in some way. Included here are divorce, separation, desertion, incarceration of the parent, placement in foster care, and single-parenting. The natural death of a parent does not appear to result in the loneliness, anger, and resentment that the other forms of family unit dissolution do.

Research has shown that, if a child is living with one parent by age sixteen, that child is seventy-percent more likely to have a criminal conviction by age fifteen, two times as likely to leave high school without a diploma, twice as likely to have a child as a teenager, fifty-percent more likely to be unemployed at age twenty, be more likely to get divorced, and be more likely to die young (Layard, 2005). Children clearly appear to need both parents (Popenoe, 1996). If one is a single parent, it may be helpful to include a relative or friend as a second-parent substitute. For example, if a child has been deserted by her or his father, perhaps the mother's brother would be available to spend some time with the child, as she or he grows up. The need for two parents is true for both heterosexual and homosexual family units.

A second important way in which attachments are disrupted is by growing up in a dysfunctional family where, by definition, the parents stay together but are not providing optimal care. There are many sources of family dysfunction and all of them may negatively impact the child in the home. Physical or sexual abuse of any family member by any family member, substance use, pathological gambling, severe and derogatory oral/verbal abuse, severe financial debt, unemployment or underemployment, and extreme social isolation by the family unit are some of the forms of severe life-stress that can overwhelm the coping resources of a family unit and lay the groundwork for a violent child later on. Again, in both disrupted and dysfunctional families, the important capacity for empathy may not be taught. Finally, the absence of a prosocial peer group and disrupted attachments at school or in the neighborhood are additional ways in which a child's attachments may become disrupted. Paradoxically, it is this loss of more normal attachment network that leads some children to join gangs, as will be seen in this chapter.

Reasonable Mastery. One of the important tasks of childhood is to acquire coping skills for life from your parents and other adult role models. Children need to learn the personal self-care skills of proper nutrition and exercise, stress management, money management, and self-soothing skills in the midst of distress. Reasonable mastery skills also include one's interpersonal skills. These skills include being able to identify correctly your own feelings (e.g., being angry and not realizing it), having empathy for others, sharing with others, and using verbal-conflict resolution skills to solve conflicts and disagreements. These personal and interpersonal skills need to be coupled with basic academic achievement to establish one's place in society.

Meaningful Purpose. Success in one's attachments to others and the development of the necessary mastery skills to be successful in life lead to prosocial values and meaningful contributions to the good of society. The absence of these skills often results in the anti-social values that are listed in table 2 in chapter 2: values such as dominance over others, revenge, jealousy, despair, and peer acceptance for gang membership.

Serious Warning Signs

The serious warning signs include depression with possible suicidal behavior, substance use disorders, and untreated PTSD. These issues have been covered in detail in previous chapters. When these issues were discussed earlier, they were in the context of troubled adults. It is important to emphasize that a child of fourteen could be overwhelmed by all three of these serious signs as well and be without the caring attachments and mastery skills necessary to resolve them. When this happens, in many cases anger erupts and violence or crime follows in the form of an urgent warning sign.

Urgent Warning Signs

The Urgent Warning Signs are the signs associated with Conduct Disorder, which is defined as violent and criminal behavior in a child before age fifteen. Included here are various forms of violence to person or property, deceitfulness and lying, failure to conform to social norms, and the emergence of moral depravity.

The 17th-century poet John Donne was wrong when he wrote that no man is an island. Many of the children in our society are islands. They do not have caring attachments and the absence for those attachments results in not learning adaptive coping skills. These prosocial-skill deficits hurt both the child and society as a whole. We have repeatedly focused on the difficulties that arise in the absence of caring attachments and noted the long-term negative impact of untreated PTSD that emerges from one's being personally victimized. Many violent youth bear both of these burdens. They are islands and angry at being treated so poorly at the hands of others.

The result is often truncated moral development; fatalism; a sense of the need for jungle survival; no empathy for others, including one's victims; and potential psychological identification with the aggressors. Both our young and our society bear a heavy price for not attending to the many signs of youth violence.

Youth Gangs

Having examined the theories of violence, the role of the core group of offenders, and the warning signs of youth violence, it is important to consider another important aspect of youth violence: its perpetration by gang members. With the possible exception of rural school shootings and some forms of affluent violence committed by individuals acting alone, much youth violence continues as a function of gang activities. As J. Bowlby points out (1982), the need for human interaction and caring attachments appears to be a given at birth and manifests itself in different ways over the lifespan. Joining a group during adolescence is one of those manifestations.

The adolescent group provides a support group for teenagers in the transition from family life to adult independence. These groupings offer skills in problem-solving, emotional support, a sense of belonging, relief from boredom, and enhanced self-esteem, among other factors. However, the research on youngsters who become violent suggests that destroyed or dysfunctional family life, the absence of caring attachments, the lack of reasonable, prosocial mastery skills, and antisocial worldviews does not in any way result in normal prosocial skills and values. Yet the social need to belong is innate and present in these troubled youngsters just as it is in their more normally adjusted peers. Unfortunately, when these dysfunctional young adults form an adolescent group, they do not develop the skills and resources to function in more prosocial ways.

The end result is a group that does not provide the nurturing support found in more intact adolescents and a group that evolves into an antisocial gang whose rules are harsh and unremitting. To demonstrate one's commitment to the group and its rules, the applicant must often commit a violent act. This act may include rape or murder. If accepted into the gang, the initiation rights are themselves violent and victimize the new member. The initiate proceeds to commit illegal and violent activities. The gang functions in many cases as a tight-knit, paramilitary group. The member knows that he or she often faces permanent disability or death, if he or she ever tries to leave.

Gang life, for all of its bravado, is grim. Many male members do not expect to live past thirty-years of age. Many are imprisoned and have severe substance use and general health problems. The outcomes for female members are no better. They too develop substance use disorders, are frequently victims of physical or sexual abuse by gang members, and often find themselves abandoned single-mothers with no resources, again by age thirty.

Types of Gangs

There are both male and female gangs and there are a variety of gang structures, which are summarized below. Deborah Prothrow-Stith (1991) has outlined these various types of gangs and the interested reader is directed to her work.

TABLE 2. Types of Gangs

Male Gangs	Scavenger Gang
	Territorial Gang
	Corporate Gang
Female Gangs	Auxiliary Gang
	Independent Gang

Table 2 presents an outline of the various types of youth gangs. There are three types of male gangs: scavenger, territorial, and corporate, and two types of female gangs: auxiliary and independent.

Male gangs. The first type of male gang is the scavenger gang. This is the most loosely organized format. It is comprised of low achievers, has no real long-term goals, has no formal structure, and changes leadership frequently. Unlike scavenger gangs, territorial gangs are organized for the specific purpose of preserving a geographical territory. These groups have members with better coping skills, include violence in their initiation rights, and expect all members to fight to the death to preserve the geographical territory from other invader gangs.

The male corporate gangs represent the highest form of socially organized gang structure. Corporate gangs exist to make a profit on some form of economic activity, such as drug dealing, prostitution, or protection monies. These gangs market to rural and urban America, and will eliminate or destroy anyone who tries to stop them or interfere in gang-business activities. Corporate-gang members are highly disciplined with strong codes of required behavior (including violence) and secrecy about the gang and its activities.

Female gangs. A common female gang is the auxiliary gang. These gangs are closely linked to the male territorial and corporate gangs, and support the criminal activities of their male peers. As in the male gangs, the use of violence to accomplish group ends is expected. Unquestionable obedience to male gang directives is routine. The second form of female gang is the independent girl gang. These independent female gangs may engage in territorial defense or in corporate business issues. They operate apart from specific male groups and have equally stringent initiation rites and codes of secret member behavior and expectations.

Life in any of these male or female gangs is harsh and there is usually no way out without outside help.

Poverty, Affluence, and Violence

Whereas the ancient Romans correctly identified that poverty was the mother of crime, what is puzzling is the rise in crime and violence in our own time by very affluent adolescents. Why would a generation of young people with the most material resources in the history of civilization murder, rob, steal, and so forth?

Part of the answer may lie in the psychology of poverty. There appear to be four basic components in the mindset of many poor persons. The first is the absence of perceptual constancy. In poor neighborhoods many things are constantly in flux. Whether you will eat, where you will live, whether you will be shot at on your way to school, whether your parent will be intoxicated in the evening may change every day. One cannot count on basic constancy in various daily life activities. This process is unsettling and can produce anxiety, depression, and anger.

The second factor is the dearth of caring attachments. Families are physically broken apart or dysfunctional. There are few good adult role-models in the neighborhood, there may not be enough teachers to have one instructor in every classroom, and there are few adult coaches for recreational teams after school. Social workers come and go. Just as there is no perceptual constancy, there is no caring attachment consistency either.

Third, in the absence of caring attachments, the poor settle on a preference for things or material goods. This choice is easily arrived at in a postindustrial state that markets all manner of goods as the answer to happiness in life, and in which consumers routinely interact with machines.

The fourth component follows quickly and logically from the first three: a pervasive fear of dependency on others. You trust no one. You have empathy for no one. You interact with no one. You remain hurt and depressed. You end up using any type of violence to obtain whatever material goods that you want. You do this because your hurt has turned to anger at being rejected and abandoned.

A similar psychological process may be at work in affluent families. To be sure, for the most part, affluent children do not have to worry about food, housing, and daily life stability. However, as their parents go off in pursuit of material goods, these children have had to ask whether their parents will be there for them after school or in the evening. Will parents be there for sports activities and birthdays? Will parents divorce as they often threaten to do? Thus, in other ways affluent children have their own form of perceptual inconstancy.

As with their poor counterparts, these affluent children may encounter the second component, that of absent caring attachments. This may come about in several ways. Parents pursuing the good life may be reluctant to parent. Parents may replace spending time with the child with giving their children money. Mother and father may not value setting limits on the child, limits that all children need. The child may be seen as a reflection of the parent's self and, thus, not accepted as an independent person with his or her own needs or strengths.

As with their less-affluent peers, these affluent children come to prefer material goods, especially cars, clothes, electronics, and drugs. They may develop a pervasive fear of dependence on others. As the affluent parents pursue the good life with its less time for childrearing, the psychologically abandoned affluent child becomes angry and depressed. In many cases these affluent children self-medicate with drugs or alcohol and, over time, this anger may erupt into violent behavioral emergencies.

Youth Homicide

This overview of youth violence concludes with a consideration of homicide and its impact on family survivors. Although young people are involved in all types of crimes and violence, homicide is becoming increasingly common among many of them.

In the industrialized world, the United States ranks among the highest in the killing of males between the ages of fifteen and twenty-four. This murder rate is occurring largely because of easily available weapons in our society and there are several reasons for these murders. Some are to control corporate drug-gang activity; some are related to drug-deals gone bad. Others are the murders of innocent persons in gang drive-by shootings; still others are murders committed during armed robberies of legitimate businesses or in home-invasions. Many more reasons could be cited but none of the reasons is an acceptable reason. The absence of caring attachments in the lives of these young assailants coupled with a history of being personally victimized and not being taught adaptive, prosocial coping skills leads to an anger that in turn has led to the death of another human being.

Individuals who survive a family member's murder have issues of their own to address. Certain factors make the murder worse and more difficult to come to terms with. Witnessing the murder makes it more difficult to accept. The relationship of the assailant to the victim may be important. Was the assailant a stranger, a neighbor, a family member? Murders that involve other crimes as well, such as sexual assault, torture, mutilation, and the like are more painful to process. Distance from the survivor's home to the murder scene, the form of death notification, the unwanted demands of the media, and dealing with the criminal justice system can all complicate bereavement.

In youth homicides, the victim loses. The assailant loses. Witnesses lose. Survivors lose. Society loses. We ignore the warning signs of youth violence at our own peril.

Specific Safety Guidelines for Youth Violence

Health-care providers are often summoned to behavioral emergencies involving youth violence. This may include murders, attempted murders, assaults and similar violent behaviors. These calls may involve the street, homes, worksites, and emergency rooms themselves.

As in the previous examples, we want to consider the type of emergency that we would need to address. Begin with the general safety guidelines first. What is the medical condition that is being reported? Check the admitting chart or call-log to see if this youth is known to the health care system. Think: scene surveillance. You will want to know the gangs present in your neighborhood and their insignias. If your scene surveillance reveals the victim to be wearing a rival gang's attire or you see some person on the street wearing rival gang attire, this is a very dangerous situation in which you may be attacked for trying to save the life of the rival gang member victim. Call for police backup. When safety is assured, remind yourself that the patient victim; the assailant, if present; witnesses; and family, friend, and neighborhood survivors will be in shock and likely operating with old brain-stem prominence. Expect potential violence from any source and use short, direct commands and responses rather than more detailed and reasoned explanations.

As you approach the patient, review the theories of violence, the early warning signs, the possible presence of substance use, and the continuum of youth warning signs. Think trauma victim as you approach the patient, trauma not only from the immediate violence but any untreated trauma from childhood that may have been triggered by the present violence. State who you are, ask permission to move closer, ask permission to provide care. State what you are going to do, so that the victim whose boundaries are shattered will not perceive your assistance as yet another attack by an assailant. Check all victims for weapons as part of a physical exam. Assume that there may be at least two other weapons on the person and check carefully for their presence. With these steps in place, use "care and cover" approach to provide necessary medical or psychiatric care.

Let us return to the burdens of both Mrs. Dalia as survivor and Jennifer as witness to homicide. The loss for Mrs. Dalia is almost beyond comprehension. Her two children were murdered, each in a year of the other on the same date. Her bereavement will be complicated by the site of the murders being in her own neighborhood. The murders did not involve additional criminal acts but her children were innocent victims, both of them. We do not know who the assailants are and we are not told the method of death notification. If the assailant turns out to be known to the family, the burden will be greater. If Mrs. Dalia learned of either or both deaths through the media or informal communication by neighbors in the street, it will likely have been even more difficult than if the police or a minister had come to the house first. We know that Mrs. Dalia already has had to deal with the media after her son's death and now will have to do this again. She will have several interactions with the legal system in the months ahead. Every visit will call forth each terrible, painful detail of her double agonies.

Jennifer, our hard-working EMS provider, is also burdened by witnessing these two deaths. She has been at the site of the murders twice and witnessed the medical aftermath of such carnage. She, too, is aware that both of these teenagers were innocent bystanders. At some level, she has sensed the fragility of life, the futility of these two deaths, and the unspeakable burden of their mother. When we, as care-providers, respond to behavioral emergencies, we want to be aware of the witnesses and survivor(s) of these emergencies as well. It is unlikely that we can attend to their needs but we can treat them with kindness and try to arrange for later community outreach. In the case of Jennifer, this includes taking care of our own as well. Table 3 summarizes the general and specific safety guidelines for responding to behavioral emergencies by violent youth.

TABLE 3. Safety Guidelines

- *Think Medical and Psychiatric Illness*
- *Think Call Log*
- *Think Scene Surveillance*
- *Think Old Brain Stem*
- *Think Early Warning Signs*
- *Think Theories of Violence*
- *Think Psychological Trauma*
- *Think Domestic Violence*
- *Think Psychiatric Emergency/Substance Use/ Suicide*
- *Think Continuum of Youth Warning Signs*

Responding to behavioral emergencies is taxing work physically and psychologically. It affects all of us, even the most dedicated and seemingly unperturbed. With our colleague Jennifer in mind, let us turn, in the last section of the book, to the implications for provider health and safety. We shall examine self-care, with strategies for self-defense and health and wellness. These are the kinds of interventions that we would want Jennifer to have had available to her at her time of crisis and available to each of us during the course of our careers, so that we remain healthy, productive, and content. Self-defense and health and wellness are important components in managing behavioral emergencies in their own right.

PART THREE

THE VIOLENT PERSON: PROVIDER SELF-CARE

SEVEN

Strategies for Self-defense

What wisdom can you find that is greater than kindness?

—Jean-Jacques Rousseau

Ellen stood beside her father in the receiving line. She was numb with grief as she stood beside the casket. Her little fourteen-year-old body would give its every ounce of energy to have those three words back

It had been a typical adolescent-parent squabble. She wanted to wear her new jersey to school the next day. Her mother thought that it was too casual for the classroom and shouting followed. In a pique of anger, Ellen yelled back at her mother, "Go drop dead!" and stormed out of the house to school. Mrs. Widner lamented the age-old wisdom that bringing up teenagers was no easy task and then headed off to work herself.

Mrs. Widner was the second-shift, nursing supervisor in the emergency room at Springfield City Hospital, a medical facility that served the city's indigent. Chronic staffing shortages made the work more difficult but she took personal satisfaction in serving these that society often overlooked. Adults with psychosis; substance use, domestic violence bruises, and advanced, untreated life-threatening medical illnesses; adolescents with unwanted pregnancies, drug overdoses, car accidents as the result of speed, and bullets from gang turf wars. Over the years, she had seen it all and yet the current level of violence seemed worse than in times past.

This increased level of violence had led Springfield City Hospital to install bulletproof glass in its emergency room.

In bay six lay a young gang member on a gurney. He had a bullet lodged in his left thigh. Campus security had warned hospital staff about checking each admission for multiple weapons, and Mrs. Widner was patting down the patient for such weapons. She found a pistol in his left front pocket, asked the patient to remove it, and then to place it on the tabletop beside him. Fearing a possible gang shoot out in the emergency room itself, she reached for the weapon. As she did so, she felt one sharp stab in her left rib cage. The adolescent had a second weapon, a knife that had been stashed in his sock. In spite of the frantic efforts of her colleagues, Mrs. Widner died almost instantly on her own emergency room floor.

"Go drop dead." I didn't mean it, Mom; I love you, Mom; I didn't mean it, thought Ellen. She approached her mother's casket and gently touched her now-stilled hand. The indestructibleness of youth had met the cold, unremitting harshness of death.

Every year several health-care providers in all disciplines, including EMS and police are killed or injured by patients attacking them with a second hidden weapon. Every year thousands of EMS and health-care providers are assaulted as they are rendering care to victims. Many others are threatened and verbally abused. Incidents such as these happen to us directly or we witness them happening to our colleagues. These events may make the work more distressing and, in time, may lead to burnout and professionals leaving the field. It need not be this way.

The work that is asked of caregivers is taxing in its own right and exposure to violence adds to the burden. However, there are things that we can do to enhance our safety and reduce our work stress as well as life-stress in general. The self-care strategies presented here, if implemented properly, will result in safety, better physical and mental health, and a meaningful sense of purpose, as we go about our work. Career growth may be enriched and lengthened, and the remaining chapters address these goals.

This chapter focuses on self-defense strategies. We have looked at general and specific guidelines for addressing the various types of behavioral emergencies. However, there is an additional set of basic safety skills for self-care that we want to know and follow on each call, so that safety is further enhanced and our work is more easily accomplished. The next chapter looks at life-stress, its role in our lives, its potential negative impact, and what we can do to reduce this life-stress and enhance our sense of well-being. Chapter 9 outlines some common examples frequently encountered by care-providers, so that we have an overview of the application of the ideas presented in this book.

Violence occurs when effective communication fails, and good communication skills are important self-defense strategies as is a knowledge of physical self-defense procedures. This chapter focuses on three aspects of self-defense: nonverbal communication, oral communication, and basic self-defense skills. This chapter is succinct but each provider will want to know that he or she is well-versed in each of these three areas. To do less is to court a heightened exposure to violence and personal harm. We begin with nonverbal communication.

Nonverbal Communication

We are always communicating. We are never not communicating with others. Even when we are asleep, we are communicating this fact to others. Individuals have two communication systems: verbal and nonverbal. Verbal communication is what we usually think of when we say someone is communicating. It refers to language and speech and what is the meaning of content of the words. However, there is a second human communication system that is even more powerful than speech. It is known as the nonverbal communication system and refers to all of the body's messages, except speech content. This includes posture, stance, attire, tone of voice, and bodily gestures about events. A person who is stooped over, dressed shabbily, and walking aimlessly communicates a different set of nonverbal messages from a neatly dressed, upright person in full stride.

It is important to remember that nonverbal behaviors have been present in humans a good deal longer than speech. The expression, "a picture is worth a thousand words," reflects this wisdom. We trust other people when their words and their nonverbal actions match most of the time and when their words and nonverbal actions are based on prosocial values. When a person's words and actions do not match, when they do not do what they say that they will do, then we do not trust that person. Because of the complexity of daily life, what a person says may not always match what he or she does. For example, someone promises to be on time but is late because of heavy traffic. These expectations should be infrequent and the explanation for the exceptions must be sound. Since nonverbal behavior has been around much longer than speech, always assume the nonverbal messages to be the more accurate barometer of intent.

Wardrobe

The way we dress is a powerful system of nonverbal communication to others about who we are and what we do. A neatly dressed professional already commands some level of respect onsite. In its own way the professional attire mitigates the potential for violence, as it is assumed that this professional has been adequately trained and knows what to do.

As noted in chapter 1, if you are not a police officer, do not dress in ways that might be misconstrued by patients and witnesses as your being a police officer. Do not wear metal badges, patches, dark blue uniforms, and have no equipment at your waist that might look like a holstered gun. This is true for both health-care providers and EMS.

Each of us additionally wants to be sure that our wardrobes and attire also enhance our safety. Begin by securing to your body anything that could be used as a weapon against you, such as a flashlight or your keys. Consider the clothing and jewelry that you may be wearing. Are you wearing anything that could be used to choke or cut you? Neckties, necklaces, high heels, earrings, hair ornaments, pierced-body jewelry, and the like may all be used as weapons against you in a struggle. Consider your hair. Could it be grabbed easily? Is it an obstacle clear to vision? In general, look the part and be sure your wardrobe does not place you at undue risk of harm.

Treatment Environments

Physical treatment environments include medical evacuation units, ambulances, emergency rooms, hospital wards, and clinic offices. These environments will appear nonverbally professional as a function of the requirements of the various regulatory agencies. However, they may still represent high-risk environments from the viewpoint of safety.

In spaces such as emergency rooms and clinic offices, desks and table work areas should be to the side against a wall near the exit door. Any chairs should be on wheels so that a quick exit from the room is possible, if the need presents itself. Desk and tables should not be in the center of treatment spaces with the care-provider on one side of the desk and the patient on the other side. In such circumstances, the patient or client can push the desk to the wall and pin the caregiver so that the caregiver is rendered helpless.

As with personal wardrobe attire, any object in the treatment areas that can be used as weapons needs to be secured. For example, paintings on the wall ought to be secured to the wall so that they cannot be used as weapons. Similarly, objects on desks such as glass trays, glass lamps, staple guns, telephone receivers, and the like need to be removed or secured. Although small working spaces, medivac units and ambulances also need to be secured so that no object or piece of medical equipment could be used as a weapon.

Posture

Our body posture communicates a good deal of information to others about our sense of self and our view of others. Consider the message from the police officer, EMS, or care-providers whose stance is intimidating, whose arms are folded, who stares at the other person, and who speaks derogatory comments in a sarcastic tone of voice. This is essentially what culture views as macho or machismo behavior. Macho may feel like power but macho may also get you killed. Patients feel that they are being demeaned. Effective communication has been lost and violence may erupt as an outcome.

The same sense of authority but without the implication of demeaning others may be had by standing straight, arms to one's sides in a relaxed stance that leaves the personal space of others intact. Moving quietly and decisively onsite permits caregivers to remain in control of the incident without increasing the risk of violence. Maintain eye contact and do not touch anyone without permission, unless it is an absolute imminent crisis.

Tone of Voice

In addition to wardrobe and posture, one's tone of voice is another form of nonverbal communication that can enhance safety. How one speaks to an issue or a medical problem can be as important as what is actually said. A tone of voice that is relaxed, soft, clear, and in measured cadence may be quieting and reassuring, as it connotes a sense of authority and competence. One's tone of voice carries more authority if it is supportive and empathic. When there is the need to set limits, firm, direct, deliberate instructions in a reasoned voice are effective and defuse potentially violent behavioral emergencies without struggle. All of these forms of nonverbal communication can be in place to enhance safety before a word is ever spoken.

Verbal Communication

In one of his plays, Shakespeare penned the following line: "Speak that I may know you." This line reflects the power of the spoken word to communicate one's thoughts and feelings in a way that can shape the worldviews and responses of others. Care-providers will always want to choose their words carefully to both enhance communication and to diminish the potential for retaliatory violence by the other party. There are some general principles of verbal communication that may prove helpful in various situations:

1. Do not use first names without permission
2. Do not argue with the patient
3. Use gentle empathic words to encourage the patient to speak freely

4. Ask broad-based or general questions to encourage information sharing
5. When possible, develop an alliance, so that you are an ally
6. Encourage the patient to describe the incident and any relevant past history
7. Involve the patient in your interventions onsite to begin to restore mastery
8. Provide any information that you may have about the event or incident to the patient
9. Formulate a plan of action with the patient's involvement in specific steps
10. Summarize the plan for the patient

In this process, do not assume that a quiet patient is coping adequately. Such persons may be severely depressed, suicidal, or in a state of psychological shock. Mitchell and Reznik (1981) cover this process in greater detail.

Verbal De-escalation

If the patient is showing any of the early warning signs of loss of control (table 4 in chapter 1), it is best to calm down the patient verbally, if this is possible.

First, leave the individual personal space. Next, stand at a forty-five-degree angle to the person. Face-to-face positioning is more likely to be perceived as threatening and lead to violence. Third, assume that the person in crisis is functioning with old brain-stem prominence and that you will need initially to utilize nonverbal modes as the primary way of communicating with the victim. Then, utilize the verbal communication steps outlined above.

Use a calm tone of voice and validate the patient's feelings. Develop an alliance, encourage the person to take some responsibility, and, then, together develop alternatives to solve the issue without resorting to violence. Keep the person talking, model calm behaviors, be at eye-level, and continuously remind the patient of nonviolent alternatives. If for safety or medical reasons you need to touch the person, ask permission to do so, explain in advance what you are going to do, and continue to explain the process as you proceed through it.

Alternative to Restraint

In tandem with the verbal de-escalation process, caregivers would do well to explore with the patient some common alternatives that have been of assistance in calming others in similar states of distress. Ask your patient what has worked in the past to help the person to calm down. Your suggesting the following strategies may prod the person's memory or expand his or her awareness of what might be helpful. Agitated persons have found these following strategies to be of assistance in calming down: talking; problem-solving; taking a walk or smoke break; listening to music; drawing; sitting quietly; using humor; and reducing sensory stimulation by distancing oneself from a level of noise, numbers of people, or the pace of activity. If the person identifies any of these strategies as potentially helpful, assist the patient to implement his or her choice of strategy, subject to whatever level of observation that you consider necessary.

Restraints

Restraints are used only to ensure safety and only when the patient presents as an imminent risk of harm to self or others. With patients restraints may not be used to restrict freedom in the absence of imminent harm and are never to be used as punishment. The imposition of restraints is a serious intervention with increased risk for violent outbursts. Patient and health-care-providers are at risk for serious injury in restraint procedures and many employee injuries occur during restraint initiatives.

There are several systems of restraint procedures. Many have different assumptions and different holds. It is important that each agency select the restraint system that seems best suited to its needs and that they train every employee and every new hire in this one system to avoid employee-team members from working at cross-purposes during restraint procedures. This decreases the risk of injury for the patient and the employees. Employees and new hires may have had previous training in some other systems of restraint. It is important that they are re-trained in the agency's system, and that they use only the agency system when providing services for that agency.

When using restraint procedures, be mindful of possible medical complications in the patient, such as past spinal-cord injuries or arthritic conditions in the elderly. Do not kneel on the person's upper back or chest as this may cause positional asphyxiation. The person's difficulties in breathing may appear as if the person is continuing to struggle but they are choking to death. It takes five employees to restrain safely – one to hold each limb and one to hold the head. Four persons may suffice, if all four employees monitor the patient's head. Two persons should not try to restrain a person. Call for police or agency back-up staff.

At times, the patient may engage in dangerous or bizarre behaviors that may frighten us. At times like these, the best of care-providers may resort to black humor, sarcasm, or forms of patient denigration, known as the stigmatizing that we mentioned earlier. All forms of stigmatization may result in patient loss of caring

TABLE 1. Communications Systems

Nonverbal Communication

- Wardrobe
- Treatment Environment
- Posture
- Tone of Voice

Verbal Communication

- De-escalation
- Alternatives to Restraint
- Restraints
- *Stigma*

attachments, reasonable mastery, and a meaningful purpose in life with the care-provider teams. As we have seen, these disruptions in the domains of good physical and mental health complicate the work to which we are asked to respond. It is in our own best interests as well as the self-esteem of our patients for us to discuss our fears with colleagues and to avoid stigmatizing onsite those that we are there to assist. Table 1 outlines the communication issues in which we want to be proficient.

Nonviolent Self-defense Releases

Although police have the needed skills, training, and legal sanction to use controlled violence where necessary, care-providers should also be trained in some system of nonviolent self-defense for use in behavioral emergencies in which violence is imminent or has occurred. Whereas the police are authorized to use controlled violence proportional to the threat, caregivers are not authorized to do so and need some system for self-protection. Most jurisdictions and agencies permit the use of some system of nonviolent self-defense (NVSD).

There are many differing systems of NVSD. Since most police and caregivers work in teams, each agency will need to select one system of NVSD. The agency will need to train all of the employees in that system, so that team members in the field are not working at cross-purposes when confronted by violent behavior.

Let us review some common NVSD releases. These are presented for illustrative purposes only. They are not meant to constitute formal training and should not be utilized by the reader in the absence of formal training in NVSD by one's agency. The author is not liable for the reader's use of these releases. Additional agency training is mandatory for each employee to be skilled in utilizing NVSD procedures.

NVSD releases emphasize flexible body posture, full body force, rotating away from the patient force, and using natural body exits through the weakest point where the fingers or hands meet. Always continue to talk to the person. Ask what is causing him or her to be angry. Ask why they are assaulting you. Ask what would help to relieve the stress and stop the violence. Pay attention to the person's natural body weapons (2 arms, 2 legs, and one head). Never intend to harm the person and always call for staff assistance. The illustrative examples below are from the Massachusetts Department of Mental Health *System of Nonviolent Strategies and De-escalation* (2002).

1. Wrist Release. When the patient has reached straight across to grasp your wrist, rotate your wrist so that the thinnest portion of your wrist can move through the thumb and finger of the patient, the natural exit. When a patient has grabbed your wrist by reaching across his or her midline, open your hand, rotate your wrist to its thinnest portion between the patients thumb and fingers. Then reach over the patient's wrist, grasp your own hand, pull your hands to your chest and step away.
2. Hand Grabs. For a simple grab, pin your own clothing. With your other hand, put your palm to the patient's palm and push patient's hand away. For a two-hand grab, weave your dominant hand over the patient's closest forearm and under the other forearm. Move your other hand up, palm-to-palm with your dominant hand. Bring the elbow of your dominant arm down to your ribcage, while pushing upward with your nondominant hand.
3. Choke Holds. Frontal Choke – use the weave intervention discussed above for two-hand grabs. Choke from rear – keep your hands in front of you, walk away from the patient while rotating your upper body back and forth at the shoulders.
4. Punch or Kick. With both hands, palms up, thumbs in, fingers together, sweep the punch or kick away. Protect your vital organs and vulnerable body parts by turning your lower body at a 45-to-90 angle to the aggressor.
5. Bites. Do not pull the bitten part from the patient's mouth. Forcefully press the bitten body part into the patient's bite.

These few release examples illustrate how NVSD interventions may provide self-protection in ways that do not harm the patient. NVSD interventions may become increasingly complex, as behav-

TABLE 2. Basic Trainings

System of Nonviolent Self-defense
Scene Surveillance
Early Warning Signs of Loss of Control
Psychological Trauma and Posttraumatic Stress Disorder
Nonverbal Communication
Verbal Communication and De-escalation Procedures
Alternatives to Restraint
Restraint Procedures
Anger Management Skills
Verbal/Oral-conflict Resolution Skills

ior escalates out of control. Again, the use of NVSD releases requires detailed training by a skilled expert in the system your employer has selected.

Table 2 outlines a basic set of trainings that will enhance employee safety and the quality of care provided by those employees to victims in behavioral emergencies. These trainings, along with the various general and specific safety guidelines, should also improve the cost-effectiveness of the services provided. These various trainings preclude or contain violence and should result in fewer incidents, less medical expense, less use of sick leave, less use of industrial accident claims, less permanent or temporary disability, sustained productivity, and improved work force morale.

This concludes the overview of the various safety strategies that caregivers may employ to protect themselves, their patients, and bystanders (cf. table 3). In behavioral emergencies, look first at the general safety guidelines that include thinking about the nature of the medical or psychiatric emergency that has been called in and examining the case log for possible helpful information about the type of call on the patient. Next, follow the general guidelines for scene surveil-

TABLE 3. Safety Guidelines

Safety

Think Medical and Psychiatric Illness
Think Call Log
Think Scene Surveillance
Think Old Brain Stem
Think Early Warning Signs
Think Theories of Violence
Think Psychological Trauma
Think Domestic Violence
Think Psychiatric Emergency/Substance Use/ Suicide
Think Continuum of Youth Warning Signs

Self-care

Think Self-defense

lance, old brain-stem prominence, the early warning signs of loss of control, and the theories of violence. Then, review the specific safety guidelines for psychological trauma, domestic violence, psychiatric emergencies, and youth violence as they may apply. In each of these potential behavioral emergencies, note the presence of untreated PTSD, and examine the potential of untreated PTSD as a contributing factor to violence in the behavioral emergency, independent of other medical or psychiatric issues. Finally, review basic personal and environmental safety issues that we would want to routinely incorporate in our professional practices.

In spite of all of this, we are at the same risk of violence as Mrs. Widner, the nurse at Springfield City Hospital. Here was a highly trained, highly experienced professional who had responded to several behavioral emergencies over the years in this emergency room. Yet in one moment one oversight resulted in death. How could this happen? Multitasking, staff shortages, preoccupation with personal or family issues, force of habit, a momentary distraction – any of these may lead one to overlook the warning signs and the necessary guidelines. It is important to look. If this is the four hundredth time you have been on a similar call, it is always important to look. If we don't look for it, we won't see it and that may be the very call that results in our being caught off guard.

Complacency, no matter how skilled the caregiver, has no place in responding to behavioral emergencies.

Our work is fascinating and rewarding but, as our summary indicates, it is also very stressful. Add to these work stresses those of everyday life and we have the potential for increased anxiety, depression, and physical illness. In some, it may lead to early retirement or a desk job. In others, it may lead to divorce, estrangement from one's children, or self-medication with drugs or alcohol. It does not have to be this way. The stresses of life and careers can be managed by means of the stress management techniques noted in the next chapter.

EIGHT

Strategies for Health and Wellness

Don't let your heart grow numb. Stay alert. It is your soul that matters.

—Albert Schweitzer

Psychologist Sarah Smith sat by the window in Seat 28A, held the small wooden box closely in her lap, and watched the sunset. How ironic and painfully sad, she thought, that they were at last together again.

There was no doubt that the man in her life was a brilliant historian. A naturalized U.S. citizen who specialized in the Civil War, he had written ten books and was a much sought-after lecturer around the world. Fame and wealth had followed.

In the beginning, however, they were young, they were foolish, and they were very much in love. From the beginning, she had pledged quietly to herself to love him forever, to help him in any way that she could. He was the center of her life.

Thus, she found it hard several years later when he suddenly asked her for a divorce to pursue "other interests," as he had put it. With her heart heavy and in shattered pieces, she mustered the courage and the depth of love necessary to let him go. In truth, in the subsequent ten years, she had never really recovered.

The facts were clear enough. The distinguished visiting professor had been killed by a drunken driver in a crosswalk in Rome, the Eternal City. The body was removed to the morgue and cremated to await its claim by the family, as no "other interests" had come forward.

Now they were together again. Her tears fell softly on the small wooden box that held her husband's ashes. They were halfway across the Atlantic with nowhere to go. His heart was stilled and, in truth, hers was stilled as well.

Night had fallen.

Just as Mrs. Widner, the nurse in the vignette, from the preceding chapter represents all of us, so does Sarah in this chapter. Here is a busy health care professional burdened by a painful stressful life event, in this case the death of her husband after their divorce of many years and what appears to be unrequited love. Sarah is all of us in that we have work-related stress as well as suffer the slings and arrows of personal life-stress. These later events include births, deaths, graduations, illnesses, financial reversals, corrupt treatment by others, and the range of human vagaries that can inflict ourselves, our spouses, our children, our loved ones, and our neighborhoods.

This untreated life-stress can exact a heavy toll on health and well-being. Extensive research documents that untreated life-stress may increase mental distress, physical illness, and premature death. Since we can predict that our work in responding to behavioral emergencies will be stressful, and since we can also assume that we will encounter inevitable personal life-stress, we need to develop individualized programs to manage stress and reduce the potential negative impact from both.

The good news is that there are several stress management techniques that can assist us in reaching this goal. The purpose of this chapter is to outline basic interventions that will help with both work and life-stress so that we remain productive and content. There are many choices among stress management interventions. Including more of the choices will enhance your stress-resistance and these various stress-reduction techniques also permit caregivers to create their own individualized programs, based on their preferences and available time.

The Nature of Work and Life-stress

In beginning this study of how best to manage stress, it is worth considering some of its basic components: élan vital and stress overdrive, one's optional level of stimulation, and the major false assumption in our culture. Awareness of these factors will help us develop a context for our own individualized stress management programs.

Élan Vital/*Stress Overdrive*

Élan vital is a French expression for vital life force. We do not have a good English equivalent. It is best understood as the biological energy of life that energizes and drives our minds and bodies. We are each born with a certain amount of this life force. It is constantly being used as we lead our lives and we cannot save it up as we might save money in a bank. When it is all used up, we are deceased.

What we do have control of is the process of how quickly it is used up. Stress management interventions permit us to utilize élan vital most effectively, so that it lasts longer than it might otherwise if we were to expend it sooner than need be. Biologically, human beings are able to live about one-hundred-ten years. In our culture, most, of us die when we are in our seventies or eighties. Our life-styles and our life-stress have used up our élan vital too quickly and we die several years earlier than we have to.

The basic process of coping with life-stress is as follows. A stressful life event (stressor) presents itself at work, at home, and/or in the community. The person copes or responds to the stressor with one's mind and one's body, as the person seeks a solution to the issue. During this interaction, the person's physiology of stress is activated. As we have noted earlier, adrenalin is released in the person's body and becomes epinephrine. Epinephrine prepares the body to face the stressor. It tightens muscles, strengthens breathing, dilates pupils to see better, and releases cortisol in the body for energy and to increase blood clotting, should the person be injured by the stressor. Epinephrine also dampens down those systems in the body that are not necessary to solve the problem such as digestion and sexual interest.

Adrenalin becomes norepinephrine in the brain and rivets our attention to the stressor so as to enhance its resolution. If the person solves the problem, the physiology of stress shuts itself off. If the problem remains unsolved, the physiology of stress remains in overdrive (even during sleep) and élan vital is used up unnecessarily. Thus, it is always in our best interest to resolve the stressors before us or at least to develop a plan to resolve them. Both of these strategies turn off the physiology of stress and preserve the unnecessary use of élan vital. Staying in constant stress overdrive results in illness and premature death.

How does one know if he or she is using his or her élan vital wisely? Our minds and bodies give us signals. If we are using it well, we will have less anxiety and depression, less physical illness, and a sense of well-being, and other things being equal (e.g., not being killed by a drunken driver), we may live longer. If we are not using our élan vital wisely, we will have the reverse of the signals that we just outlined. For those of us who work helping other people, there is an additional interpersonal source of stress that is known as burnout. Burnout occurs when we have taxed our personal resources too heavily in assisting others. This is a helping profession problem and our minds and bodies give us messages in addition to those just noted that we are not using our élan vital wisely. The two most prominent signs of burnout are physically and psychologically withdrawing from those we are there to assist, and then verbally denigrating them. Comments such as, "all citizens lie" (police), "all students cheat" (teachers), "all patients make trouble" (health-care providers) are common examples of verbal denigration. (The reader is referred to Everly and Lating [2002] for a more detailed discussion of the human stress response.

Optimal Level of Stimulation

Our nervous systems are constructed to take in information about the world around us through our major senses of vision, hearing, taste, touch, and smell. Messages from the senses pass through the limbic system where they receive an emotional component, and then travel to the prefrontal cortex where the brain makes a decision about what to do with the information.

The flow of information from the senses comes in varying intensities. Our bodies are built to function best when the incoming sensory information is in manageable amounts. This is called our optimal level of stimulation. It is when we feel most comfortable addressing the demands of the stressors of the day. Too much sense input (overload) overwhelms us cognitively and we react with irritability and anger. Similarly, too little sense input (boredom) also leads to reactions of irritability and anger. The stress management implications of our optimal levels of stimulation are clear. If one is overwhelmed, one needs to reduce the issues being encountered. If one has too little input, one needs to increase the sense input.

However, there is one further nuance in our study of optimal levels of stimulation. People are born with different levels of sensory need (Scitovsky, 1976). Some people need very little stimulation before they reach their optimal levels of stimulation. These individuals are quiet, reflective, have a few very close friends, are interested in nature, and engage in social activities that are quieter. On the other hand, other individuals need a great deal of stimulation before they reach their optimal levels of sensory input. These persons have a great many friends, enjoy intense and crowded activities, and enjoy large parties and gatherings.

In the United States, about one-quarter of the population need less sensory stimulation and three-quarters welcome a good deal of sense input. In terms of stress management, it is important to know into which group you fall. This can be readily determined by keeping a daily log for two weeks. At the end of this time, count up the number of activities that you engaged in daily, look at their general nature, and ask yourself if they are primarily limiting or expansive sensory activities. Then, ask yourself the most important question. Was I reasonably content during these two weeks, when I was engaged in these activities, or was I feeling either bored or overwhelmed? You may find that you have been working at cross-purposes with your own body rhythms.

Cultural False Assumption: "I Can Have It All"

In a postindustrial state with its emphasis on immediate gratification through material goods, a false cultural assumption has emerged that each of us can have it all. Having it all is presented in our societal advertising as having all the accoutrements of the good life – as many houses, cars, clothes, vacations, meals, promotions, and the like. Our culture tells us there is no limit. However, from a stress-management point of view, there is a limit and that limit is called illness and death.

There is not enough time in one's day to have it all. There is not enough money in one's life to have it all. There is not enough physical energy in one's body to have it all. Most importantly, the time spent in purchasing the good life and then consuming it leaves little time for our caring attachments to others. Ours is a wealthy culture and we can have much of its resources over the course of a lifetime. However, trying to have it all, all at once, puts the body in stress overdrive and deprives us of time with our caring attachments, the very attachments that can buffer life-stress physically as well as psychologically.

Managing Work and Life-stress

We begin now to examine a number of different strategies to manage the stress of life and work and to preserve élan vital. Select those that seem appropriate to your needs and that motivate you to do them. As you master one, feel free to add another. When that is mastered, consider a third. The more strategies that you incorporate, the greater the number of resources that you will have to cope with the ups and downs of life as you go along. Do not try to do all of these all at once. That will only place you in stress overdrive and defeat the purpose of stress-management interventions. Give yourself at least six months to two years to incorporate these strategies into your daily life. Take longer, if you need to. However, you will feel better and less stressed as you go along.

Right-brain Activities

The first helpful stress management strategy is to use right-brain activities to shut off the stress response and preserve élan vital. Figure 5 of chapter 1 depicts a side view of the cortex and limbic system. The cortex is the top part of the brain that is located right beneath our skulls. If we were to adopt another view of the brain and look down on it from above, we would notice that the brain is divided into left and right brain hemispheres. Left brain is for language, thinking, and problem-solving. Right brain is for visual-spatial locomotion in the environment, so that we can move about without bumping into things and hurting ourselves. The right brain also has the remarkable capacity to shut off stress-response overdrive.

Although both sides of the brain may be active at the same time, like walking and talking simultaneously, only one sphere can be dominant at any time. Worrying occurs when the left brain is dominant and calmness may be present when the right brain is dominant. Right-brain activities reduce stress and the good thing about right-brain activities is that one cannot use right-brain activities to reduce stress, if the person is facing a true crisis. Thus, right-brain activities may be utilized daily to take the edge off of work and personal life-stress. In this way, élan vital is not dissipated unwisely.

Common right-brain activities include aerobics; brisk walking; relaxation exercises; biofeedback; prayer and meditation; humor and crying; and art, music, and dance. Some hobbies, like photography are also right-brain activities. Aerobics is the most powerful stress-reducer, and relaxation exercises are easily implemented. These two alone can greatly reduce life-stress. The appendixes include guidelines for aerobic exercise and relaxation exercises. Everyone should see his or her physician to be cleared for participation in an aerobics program. Follow any directions from your physician.

Wise Lifestyle Choices

A quarter of a century ago, Belloc and Breslow (1973) studied healthy habits that contributed to good health and sense of well-being. Their findings are as true today as when they were first published. They noted the importance of seven different lifestyle choices that preserved élan vital from unnecessary waste.

1. *No smoking.* Cigarettes contain many chemicals that may cause cancer, in addition to taxing the pulmonary and cardiovascular systems.
2. *Regular Sleep Patterns.* Our sleep cycle runs in ninety-minute intervals. During the first sixty minutes, our body repairs the wear and tear of our day's activities. During the remaining thirty minutes, our brain reviews andstores in memory the day's event. This last thirty minutes is known as REM sleep or rapid eye movement sleep. Both parts of the sleep cycle are important in our maintaining good health and functioning. Most persons need eight hours of sleep to maintain optimal health.
3. *Regular Meals/No Snacks.* America is facing an obesity epidemic due to lack of exercise and faulty eating habits. Our meals should be low in fat, low in sodium, high in fruits and vegetables, high in whole-grain breads, and low in refined white sugar. Most snack foods are high in sugar, fat, and sodium. A better snack would be a piece of fruit.
4. *Breakfast Every Day.* Our metabolisms, which digest food and burn calories, come on at four o'clock in the morning. Stomach acids are activated at that time to digest the day's food. If we do not eat breakfast, we are not providing the necessary fuel or energy to function well during the day and the acids remain in the stomach and may cause wear and tear on the stomach's lining.
5. *Moderate or No Drinking.* We have seen in chapter five how substance use disorder can impair the capacity of the mind and body of the person. The use of alcohol often results in alcoholism due to genetic predisposition, food allergies, low

blood sugar, or continuous use over time that changes the person's body cells. E. J. Khantzian's self-medication hypothesis (1977) may apply as well to us as to our patients or clients.

6. *Normal Body Weight.* We live in a sedentary age. We sit before computers, watch television, and play video games. As a nation we are becoming obese, especially our children. Obesity results in many serious medical problems, including diabetes and joint problems. We attain our normal body weight at about age twenty-two and we should strive to attain and maintain that weight.
7. *Regular Exercise.* On the phylogenetic scale, humans are considered members of the animal kingdom. Like all animals, our bodies are meant to be mobile and exercise is an important aspect of physical strength, flexibility, and general conditioning. Lack of exercise is associated with heart disease, cancer, and a loss of the sense of well-being.

These healthy habits reduce life-stress and may be easily implemented in your life at no cost over a period of six months to two years. Belloc and Breslow (1973) also note that these healthy habits were associated with the wise use of élan vital, so that élan vital was dissipated more slowly. If you are forty-five and were to do five of the seven steps noted above, you would live ten years longer than a forty-five-year-old person who did four or fewer. If you are older, it is not too late to start. If you are younger than forty-five, you may be able to extend your life beyond the ten-year period.

Stress-Resistant Persons

At one point in my professional career, I was interested in those persons who seemed to remain healthy and did not come to our hospitals and clinics. I wondered how they adjusted so well to the stressors of life. To find the answers, I began a research project that involved 1,200 persons over a twelve-year period. I studied the adult men and women in an evening college program. These students had to deal with many stresses, including working full-time, being married, rearing children, taking several courses each semester, driving to the college in rush-hour traffic in addition to whatever other personal life-stressor with which they were confronted. I sought to identify those skills that were helpful in solving life-stress with minimal impact on health and well-being. I refer to these adaptive skills as the skills of stress-resistant persons (Flannery, 2003) and they are summarized in table 1. These skills are not innate but can be learned by any of us and appear helpful to men and women, all races, all ethnic groups, and all social classes.

TABLE 1. Stress-Resistant Persons

1. *Reasonable Mastery*
2. *Personal Commitment to Task*
3. *Wise Lifestyle Choices*
   - *Few Dietary Stimulants*
   - *Aerobic Exercise*
   - *Relaxation Exercises*
4. *Social Support*
5. *Sense of Humor*
6. *Concern for Welfare of Others*

The first skill of adaptive problem solvers is reasonable mastery. Good problem-solvers clearly identify the true problem; gather information to solve it; develop a few strategies to solve the problem; implement one strategy; evaluate its effectiveness; and implement a second strategy, if the first one is not working. They also know that in life not everyone can solve every problem. They make good-faith efforts to solve problems, but, if the problem is beyond reasonable effort, they will move on to the next issue in life.

The second skill is being personally committed to some task or event in life, such as improving one's work skills, rearing one's family, completing school, participating in a community project, and the like. The task need not consume more than a few hours of the person's week, but the goal provides a meaningful purpose in life.

The third stress-resistant factor had to do with wise lifestyle choices, such as those noted by Belloc and Breslow (1973). Stress-resistant persons avoid the dietary stimulants of caffeine, nicotine, and refined white sugar; participated in aerobic exercises for at least three twenty-minute periods spread out over seven days; and engage in some form of relaxation exercises for fifteen minutes each day. Individuals knew that not engaging in these activities would make them feel out-of-sorts and less productive.

Stress-resistant persons are sociable people. They have friends consistent with their optional level-of-stimulation requirements and enjoy interpersonal contact. These adaptive problem-solvers utilize a sense of humor to see the paradoxes in life and, thus, reduce stress. Finally, they are motivated and energized by assisting others in caring endeavors. The incorporation of these skills in your personal life will result in better physical and mental health and you will enjoy life more often. As with the previous stress management techniques, it will take six months to two years to gradually incorporate these stress-resistance skills in your daily routine.

Time Management

Ours is an age of time scarcity and multitasking (Linder, 1970; Schor, 1991), and most of us want to manage our time more effectively to have more leisure, family, and rest time. The chronologist, DiGrazia (1964), may be able to help us understand where all of our time is going.

Several years ago, he pointed out the five basic ways that persons use time: work time, personal time, culture time, consumption time, and idleness. Work time refers to hours of paid employment that we may have in full-time, part-time, or paid consulting positions. Personal time refers to those activities that keep us functioning as persons. Included here are personal-care tasks such as eating, sleeping, showering, as well as managing our finances, getting the car repaired, mowing the lawn, and similar kinds of tasks. Culture time refers to time spent in participating or attending fine arts performances like going to a symphony. For most Americans, culture time is a very small part of the average person's week. Most of us spend a good deal of time on work and personal care tasks.

Consumption time is often thought of as leisure but they are not the same. Leisure time refers to a relaxed, stress-free period of time to visit with loved ones and friends, pursue hobbies, take a restful vacation, sit quietly and enjoy nature, and so forth. Consumption time, however, refers to the time that we spend consuming and using the material goods of our postindustrial state beyond those services needed for personal care tasks. In a society that overemphasizes material goods, individuals accumulate so many material goods that they have to use several of them at once to get to use them all. For example, the individual comes home from work, turns on the compact music disc or plays with the iPod, turns on the microwave, selects a frozen television dinner, turns on the television, and reads the day's newspaper all at once. Consumption takes a good deal of time and may be mentally and physically very tiring. Finally, idleness is the last category of time and it, too, is not leisure time, as we usually think of it. Idleness has a precise technical meaning: the person has no paid work time and, therefore, no money to fund consumption time.

A quick examination of these categories of time suggests why ours is an age of time scarcity. Many of us are working extra jobs to purchase more goods and services for consumption time. Instead of cutting back on consumption time in order to have more leisure, most of us cut back on personal time. We sleep less, we eat more fast-food meals, we do not exercise regularly, and our stress response stays in overdrive until we get sick. Managing time means living within our means and cutting back on consumption time. None of us can have it all.

Your Psychological Work Contract

Health-care providers need to be aware of a potential, common source of work stress. It is known as a disruption in our psychological work contract (Levinson, 1976).

When we apply for a job, we are given a printed job description of the duties and an explanation of benefits. These undoubtedly are motivators for us to perform our work well. However, there are other powerful motivators that are not listed among the materials from the company. These powerful motivators are found in what Levinson refers to as our psychological work contracts.

Our psychological work contract refers to the unwritten but conscious aspects of the work that motivate each of us personally to do our best. Each of us has a vision of what our ideal work conditions would be: what type of work, what type of setting, what type of working conditions, and what types of colleagues that would make us work our best. Table 2 presents a list of common psychological factors that motivate many people. Which are the most important ones for you in your worksite? When your company offers you work that fits the psychological components of your unwritten work contract, there is a good "fit" between the company's needs and your skills.

TABLE 2. Common Psychological Work Components

Achievement	*Personal Growth*
Career Advancement	*Personal Satisfaction*
Cutting Edge Advance in Field	*Power*
Flexible Work Hours	*Prestige/Status*
Friendship	*Socialization*
Influence Company/Government Policy	*Support Family*

Employees in all careers, including health-care providers, will experience undue stress when the company is no longer able to meet the psychological work contract needs of its employees. This is a common problem for loyal employees whose job descriptions have not changed over time. Such employees may become bored, depressed, angry, and/or demoralized. Poor company/employee fits may also arise when companies downsize, lay off members of the work force, or are bought out by a larger company. All of these sources of organizational stress can lead to poor morale and lowered productivity.

If you are unhappy at work, think about your unwritten motivators in your psychological work contract. If important motivators have been disrupted, meet with your supervisor to see if your formal job description can be rewritten to include company work that reflects your psychological work contract needs. For example, if you appreciate being on cutting-edge advances in your field and the company's reorganization has left you with a routine desk job, see if part of your work time can be redesigned to include the cutting-edge work. If the lack of "fit" continues or worsens, consider employment in another work setting, if this is possible. Regardless of your decision, know that a dispirited, angry, depressed employee whose job is not addressing important psychological needs will not be at the top of his or her skills and productivity. Reduce the source of stress by creating tasks that are meaningful and challenging at work or in your private life.

Critical Incident Stress Management

Finally, Critical Incident Stress Management (CISM; Everly and Mitchell, 2002) refers to a comprehensive set of crisis intervention procedures to assist the individual in times of critical incidents at work and in one's personal life. Individual, group, and family crisis intervention procedures are called upon to reduce and mitigate the acute psychological distress of the incident and to prevent or mitigate the onset of PTSD. These interventions are often routinely offered to our patients with helpful results. The same may be true for care-providers themselves. CISM procedures may prove to be of invaluable assistance in dealing with the psychological aftermath of violent behavioral emergencies as well as in the aftermath of personal tragedies, such as the drive-by shooting of one's own innocent child.

ASAP (Flannery, 1998) as a CISM procedures has sound empirical support and should be routinely fielded after critical incidents have occurred. Participation should be voluntary to avoid in some the recall of previous traumatic memories, the psychological taxing of individuals who already feel overwhelmed, vicarious traumatization in a group setting, and other similar reasons. Individuals with these issues can be seen on individual referral by therapists who specialize in treating victims of psychological trauma and PTSD. The Assaulted Staff Action Program (ASAP; Flannery, 1998) discussed in chapter 1 is specifically designed to assist care-providers with the psychological sequellae often experienced in the aftermath of responding to critical incidents in many types of settings, and has had proven value for over twenty years.

Table 3 presents a brief overview of the various stress management strategies that we have discussed to avoid stress overdrive with its increased risk of illness and premature death. One cannot race through acquiring stress management skills. This is the paradox. As we noted earlier, to rush through will only increase the life-stress that we are trying to reduce. Go at a reasonable pace, enjoy the process, and, in time, a sense of well-being will emerge.

TABLE 3. Health and Wellness Skills

1. *Utilize Right-Brain Activities*
2. *Make Wise Lifestyle Choices*
3. *Develop the Skills of Stress-Resistant Persons*
4. *Manage Time Wisely*
5. *Know Your Psychological Work Contract*
6. *Utilize Critical Incident Stress Management Procedures, When Indicated*

Table 4 presents a final summary of safety and self-care guidelines. We have reviewed a good deal of information but the guidelines are presented in succinct bullet format to aid in remembering the main points. The bullets are meant to alert us to possible high-risk situations and to remind us of the risk assessment and management strategies that we may need to implement. One can always

TABLE 4. Safety Guidelines

Safety

- *Think Medical or Psychiatric Illness*
- *Think Call Log*
- *Think Scene Surveillance*
- *Think Old Brain Stem*
- *Think Early Warning Signs*
- *Think Theories of Violence*
- *Think Psychological Trauma*
- *Think Domestic Violence*
- *Think Psychiatric Emergencies/Substance Use/ Suicide*
- *Think Continuum of Youth Warning Signs*

Self-care

- *Think Self-Defense*
- *Think Health and Wellness*

return to the various types of behavioral emergencies that we have discussed for a more detailed review.

To conclude the analysis of risk management strategies for safety and care, the final chapter presents case studies of some commonly encountered violent or potentially violent persons that we are called upon to serve. In each case example, the various relevant general and specific safety guidelines are noted so that we have a full overview in specific critical incidents of how to field the various assessment and risk management strategies outlined in the book as well as minimize our levels of stress.

NINE

The Guidelines in Practice: Case Examples

Look after him . . . .

—Luke 10:35

"Justice, Justice!" she had cried out as the crowd of neighbors sought to comfort her in the middle of the street. They thought she was referring to the drunken driver but she was speaking to God.

In the street lay the badly battered body of her eight-year-old son, Richard. Pieces of brain tissue were scattered about, blood spatter was everywhere. Ellen Knight had just witnessed her son being killed by a drunken driver in the crosswalk before his school. Justice. Justice. . . .

Richard's young life had been shaped by violence. His mother had run away from her own family after being repeatedly battered by her father. She was surprised and saddened to learn a few years later that she had married another violent man. He beat her before the pregnancy, he beat her during the pregnancy, and he beat her after the pregnancy. In time, he went after Richard. One evening she took Richard and herself to a battered women's shelter where she remained terrified of his threats to stalk and kill her. . . .

Overwhelmed with wordless grief, she stood beside the casket of her now-stilled little boy. Would her ex-husband come to the funeral? Would he be drunk? Would he be violent? In the darkness of the night it didn't matter anymore.

Her Richard was gone. The darkness was palpable. Justice had become a hollow void.

In this book we have noted ten safety and two self-care guide ines for health-care providers. These guidelines are to remind each of us responding to a call for assistance to scan the guidelines for each incident to assess for potential, high risk, behavioral emergency situations. If a guideline(s) appears relevant to the situation, keep in mind the various risk management strategies for safety for that situation that we have reviewed.

In each of the previous chapters, we have reviewed the relevant guidelines pertinent to the specific case example that began each chapter. Here at the conclusion of the book we shall examine the scanning process for utilizing all of the relevant guidelines pertinent to examples of frequently encountered, potential behavioral emergencies. Included are the drunken-driver manslaughter noted above as well as examples of attempted homicide/suicide, youth violence, and the impaired functioning of a colleague at work. These examples by no means exhaust the list of all possible behavioral emergencies. However, each is illustrative of how to use the safety guidelines to scan each type of incident quickly. As we shall see, the scanning process is similar in all behavioral emergencies, so that the cases presented are in fact also preparing us to approach any behavioral emergency safely. Again, if a guideline(s) appears relevant in any given incident, we will want to review and utilize the relevant risk management strategies associated with that guideline(s).

Case Example 1: The Sudden, Violent Death of a Child

Ten-year-old Richard, described above, lies deceased in the street. The drunken driver did not flee and is being detained by the neighbors, until police arrive on the scene. Richard's mother, a victim of past domestic violence, is also in the street and is being calmed by other neighbors. She is clearly and understandably very distraught. If we were asked to assist Richard's mother onsite as a mental health crisis outreach team, how would we utilize the safety guidelines to help us?

First, we would need *to think* about the presence of any *medical or psychiatric illness* before we arrive. What conditions might be present in Richard's mother? Conditions to consider would be depression with possible suicidal thoughts or behaviors, possible untreated PTSD from the present incident, as well as the past repeated domestic violence. We would want to make a note to ask her about other possible medical conditions that she may have, when the opportunity presents itself. What conditions may be present in the driver? Obviously, substance use is present, but did the driver sustain any head injuries in this accident? Is the driver depressed and suicidal both as a result of this accident and as a side effect from using alcohol? Is the driver's substance use secondary to a hypoglycemic condition? All of the conditions noted here are medical/psychiatric illnesses known to be associated with the risk of violence, and we will need to monitor the scene for any potential of violence from these conditions. This situation is a behavioral emergency with several risks for violence.

Next, we would want *to think call log and/or patient's admitting chart*. Has the agency had any previous contacts with the deceased son, the mother, this family, the driver, or this neighborhood generally? In past emergency runs or in previous visits to the health care facility, have any of these people been involved in behavioral emergencies with us that led to violence or attempted violence? If the answer is "yes," then heightened concern for safety is in order as we provide care to the principals.

Think scene surveillance is always necessary in any incident and is no less true in this case. Can we initially view the scene from a distance to familiarize ourselves with the incident? Can we account for all or most of the persons on the street? Where are the identified victims? Have the police arrived as yet? Is anyone behaving violently as we arrive? Are any weapons visible? As we park, have we left ourselves an escape route, if one is needed?

The next guideline is very relevant to this incident. We need to *think old brain stem.* The death of a child, a drunken driver, a distraught mother, and several angry neighbors should lead us to assume that many of these individuals may have been overwhelmed, will be responding by old brain stem prominence, and will not be fully utilizing the powers of pre-frontal cortex higher reasoning. We will retain this assumption until conditions indicate otherwise.

Because of possible old brain stem functioning, guideline five, assumes greater importance than might otherwise be the case. *Think early warning signs* of loss of behavioral control, when you arrive onsite. Continuously monitor those in tenuous control specifically and everyone at the scene in general. Survey the appearance and behaviors of Richard's mother and any angry neighbors, as your interventions proceed.

Think theories of violence and review in your own mind what might explain this act of violence by the driver. Culturally, this incident is occurring in the present age of anomie with its de-emphasis on concern for the welfare of others. Biologically, the substance use of alcohol appears to be a major contributing factor. Additional medical and psychiatric issues in the driver remain to be assessed. Sociologically, substance use also appears to be a contributing factor; but other possible sociological factors such as the aftermath of domestic violence, inadequate schooling, or discrimination will need to be evaluated. From a psychological standpoint, we know the driver does not handle life-stress well and has issues with reasonable mastery. We do not know his reason for drinking at present, although he may be using the alcohol to self-medicate anxiety. Richard's mother is biologically depressed, is likely a victim of untreated PTSD, and sociologically is a victim of domestic violence. Psychologically, she is feeling no sense of personal mastery or control of her life and is very angry at life treating her so unfairly.

The basic message to those of us attempting to provide care is that any number of the theories of violence are likely present and all are associated with brain disinhibition of cortical control. Therefore, the likelihood of violent outbursts should be expected and we should monitor the various etiologic factors for possible loss of control.

Guidelines seven through ten refer to specific psychological situations associated with potential violence in these behavioral emergencies. In the incident before us, we will want to *think psychological trauma.* Richard's mother may be traumatized by witnessing the death of her son, and the driver and neighbors who may have witnessed the accident also may be traumatized. In addition, we know that Richard's mother has a past history of domestic violence and neighbor witnesses may also have past trauma histories. Since there is no imminent life-threatening medical emergency, we will want to approach the principals and the neighbors, as if they were trauma victims until we learn otherwise. We would want to use the specific risk management steps of chapter three: observing boundaries, clarifying who we are, explaining what we need to do, and so forth.

In this case we also want to *think domestic violence.* Even though we are not going into a home, we have a victim in the street with a history of domestic violence, as the neighbors have told us. Although safety from her domestic assailant does not appear to be of concern, she is a victim of domestic violence and we need to follow the risk management strategies from chapter 4, for victims. Many of these are similar to those of trauma victims.

From the case example, it is clear that we need to *think psychiatric emergencies/substance use/suicide.* Richard's mother is likely seriously depressed and may become both psychotically depressed and suicidal during your time with her. Substance use is also present in the driver and neighbor witnesses may also become depressed and suicidal. In this example, we would want to follow the specific risk management strategies for these medical conditions: assessing suicide-risk, monitoring withdrawal effects from substances, evaluating the needs for psychotropic medications, and so forth.

Unless the driver turns out to be a youth or gang member, we do not need to *think continuum of youth warning signs.* The guidelines for self-care, *think self-defense* and *think health and wellness,* pertain to the well-being of care-providers and will be explored in the last case example, of the impaired professional.

We have now walked ourselves through the safety guidelines for the behavioral emergency. Our review of the bullets suggests which risks for violence might be present, how to understand their etiologies, and what risk management strategies for safety we would need to implement as we go about our work of assisting the victim. As noted earlier, no one can predict violence with one hundred percent accuracy, but the overview of risk that we have arrived at as we reviewed the guidelines should help to reduce the risk of violence, enhance safety, and improve the quality of the services that we provide.

In the present case, the crisis intervention team under the direction of a psychiatrist did a thorough scene analysis and correctly concluded that no weapons were present, and that the principles and neighbors in the street were angry or frightened but in control. Richard's mother had no other major medical problems that might result in an additional behavioral emergency in the street. However, the family was known to the police because of several domestic violence calls, and it was likely that she might be a victim of untreated PTSD from her son's sudden death and her years of domestic violence. The health care staff maintained clear boundaries with her, proceeded slowly to assist her, and explained each step (e.g., the need to move her away from her son's body when the coroner arrived). Since she was initially functioning in old brain stem mode, they were especially gentle and repetitive in their simple communications with her, until her higher brain functioning returned. She was not acutely suicidal or homicidal, so they began first to provide grief counseling. Richard's mother stood by her son's body, and would not leave the scene until her son had been removed. The crisis team honored her request and comforted her emotionally during the wait.

The driver was hopelessly intoxicated and could not communicate clearly. He was arrested and taken to a shock trauma unit for medical evaluation and detoxification. The police stood guard at the hospital.

When Richard's body had been removed, family members took his mother home. They had the crisis team hotline number and were instructed to call for any reason.

The crisis team then held a small group meeting for any of the neighbors who wished to share what they had been through. Each was also given the hotline number for future need.

This behavioral emergency had several potential sources for violence, but the intervention team, following the safety guidelines that we reviewed, and employing the needed risk management strategies, were able to complete their important clinical work without any violent, vengeful outbursts.

Table 1 presents the safety/self-care guidelines assessment/intervention tool, to serve as a reminder of what potential sources of violence may be present in any particular call, and what risk management strategies will benefit from review before arriving onsite.

TABLE 1. Safety Guidelines Assessment/Risk Management Tool

Guidelines	*Issue Relevant to Call for Assistance*	*Assessment/Risk Management Strategies to be Reviewed*
Safety		
Think Medical or Psychiatric Illness	X	
Think Call Log	X	
Think Scene Surveillance	X	X
Think Old Brain Stem	X	X
Think Early Warning Signs	X	X
Think Theories of Violence	X	
Think Psychological Trauma	X	X
Think Domestic Violence	X	X
Think Psychiatric Emergencies/ Substance Use/Suicide	X	X
Think Continuum of Youth Warning Signs		
Self-care		
Think Self-defense		
Think Health and Wellness		

This tool can be in paper (or electronic) format as outlined here and may be a helpful mnemonic device. It can be reduced to wallet size and carried on one's person at all times. Its importance is that it emphasizes the need to review these materials in each case. An individual health-careprovider and/or team would check off any relevant safety guideline bullet and similarly check off any set of risk management that may be relevant. Table 1 is filled out as the crisis intervention team responding to the fatal car accident would have completed it. An *x* indicates potential risks to be assessed and associated risk management strategies to be reviewed.

Case Example 2: Attempted Murder/Suicide

A local community mental health clinic offers emergency outreach services and will go with the police, when necessary, to deal with behavioral emergencies. It is directed by the chief social worker. One Wednesday afternoon, its emergency services staff received a call from the police for assistance. A woman had called in a panic because her forty-year-old husband suddenly began holding a knife to their infant son's throat and threatening to kill the baby or himself. No other information was available.

As the clinical care staff waited for their police escort, they began the review of the safety guidelines, a review that was the standard operating procedure of the clinic in all potentially high-risk behavioral emergencies.

Think medical or psychiatric illness. The staff began to review possible medical conditions that might lead to such apparent impulsive rage. Delirium, glycemic conditions, intracranial bleeding, a traumatic head injury, psychosis, depression, domestic violence, substance use, and untreated PTSD were some of the conditions that they considered. In case of a physical medical problem, the police would be with them for hospital transport and paramedic services could be summoned immediately.

Think call log. The staff next considered whether the patient and/or the family were known to them or the police. Neither agency had any information about this family.

Think scene surveillance. The staff would ask the police for transport without sirens and to survey the house and street for anything askew. No one knew if this was a domestic violence call. The wife had told the police that it was not domestic violence but victims are not always accurate reporters.

Think old brain stem. The crisis team has made an assumption that the father was in old brain stem functioning and that they would approach him slowly with short repetitive words to restore higher brain functioning. They intended to operate very slowly to minimize any impulsive stabbing of the child. They would attempt to talk the father down and wait him out for however long might be necessary. His wife appeared to have higher cognitive functioning, when she called the police, but she would be evaluated as well.

Think early warning signs. In the present case, the early warning signs had already been present, when the original call for assistance was made. Onsite, his wife would be assessed and monitored in case the stress of the present crisis has resulted in maladaptive coping on her part, since the time her call was made.

Think theories of violence. This father lives in an era of cultural anomie with its license to impinge on the rights of others, including infants. Biologically, the father might have any number of physical medical problems as noted earlier, including intracranial bleeding, hypoxia due to cardiac illness, and renal disease. From a psychiatric point of view, he could be psychotic, seriously depressed, abusing substances, and the like. Sociologically, this might be a case of domestic violence but little was known of this family. Clearly, the father is psychologically out of control. Murdering one's child is not an adaptive solution to a life crisis. What would make him so angry that he would want to murder his own child? No one knew at this point.

Think psychological trauma and *think domestic violence.* The team has already made a note to evaluate for the presence of these issues.

Think psychiatric emergencies/substance use/suicide. Clearly, the team was dealing with a possible suicide. Whether this was due to psychiatric illness and/or substance use would be an obvious area of inquiry.

Think continuum of youth warning signs. Youth violence did not appear to be part of the presenting problem.

Psychological trauma, domestic violence, psychiatric emergencies, substance use, and suicide each called for specific risk management strategies for approaching the patient, the distraught father. His wife might be a helpful source of information in ruling any or all of these issues in or out. In concert with the police, the team devised the following strategy. The police would enter first. If there was no domestic violence occurring, the police would stand in the back of the room. The crisis team would follow. One member would meet and debrief the wife. The others would speak to the husband from a distance to engage him without his feeling trapped. The immediate goal was to secure the weapon before it was used on either father or son.

And the outcome? The scene surveillance went as planned due to sound training in how to approach such a house call. The collective strategy to assist the father also proceeded smoothly as planned. The police were a quiet but clear presence. The man's wife confirmed that there had been no psychological trauma, domestic violence, or substance use in their marriage and she had no evidence that her husband was psychotic, when the signs and symptoms were explained to her.

The team approached the father very slowly, employed the steps to restore higher reasoning, and found a distraught, recent legal immigrant, who had little schooling and command of English, who had experienced repeated forms of discrimination in this country, and had just been laid off from his job. He was overwhelmed emotionally and financially. The job loss occurred three months after the birth of his son and in the midst of a midlife crisis. He did not want to kill his son but felt the son should not have to experience the life that he had gone through to date.

In time, the father put the knife down and was discreetly searched for any additional weapon(s). There were none and he was transported to the hospital for safety, care, and a thorough medical and psychiatric work-up. The police were dispatched and the hospital's home visiting team was contacted and arrived onsite to provide care to mother and son. At that point, the crisis intervention team returned to the hospital.

Again, by following the safety guidelines and utilizing the respective risk management strategies as indicated, the police and the crisis team had averted a possible death and precluded any other aggressive outbursts. In providing care, they had ensured everyone's safety, including their own. For practice, it may be helpful to fill out the safety guidelines assessment/intervention tool in table 1 for this case example.

Case Example 3: Youth Violence

The call came in at 11:10 P.M. A young gang member had been shot in the thigh in a drive-by shooting. He was in the street at the corner of Elm and Grove Avenues and he was bleeding profusely. Paramedics Mike and Kevin knew the neighborhood well. Crime-infested, poverty-stricken, saturated with drugs, the Wells Place Housing Project was the most dangerous section of the city. Rival gangs continually fought block by block for both territory and drugs customers. Even the police always went in twos and often in fours. A fellow paramedic was nearly killed in the same area last summer in broad daylight as he tried to provide care to a similar shooting victim in a nearby park. A rival gang member did not want the shooting victim to survive and shot at the paramedic to prevent lifesaving care from being administered. This call had come in the nighttime and would be a potentially very dangerous behavioral emergency.

Michael and Kevin began to review the safety guideline bullets and the attending relevant risk management strategies that might need to be fielded.

Think medical and psychiatric illnesses. They were already aware of the gunshot wound with the potential severing of an artery. Hypovolemia (massive bleeding) and/or possible hypoxia (lack of oxygen) due to secondary cardiac or respiratory complications were at times associated with gun shooting. Kevin and Mike would certainly want to be aware of substance use, as it was well known that both gangs used and sold cocaine regularly. They would need to assess for withdrawal side effects and possible psychosis due to cocaine poisoning. Crashing from cocaine in withdrawal was associated with violent outbursts as well. Other possible medical and psychiatric illnesses could be assessed, after they had removed the victim to their medivacuation unit and were safely away from the scene.

Think call log. Although they were not given the name of the victim, their unit had had several calls to assist members of both gangs. These calls were always dangerous and the paramedics learned the insignias and codes of both gangs and always employed a "care and cover" approach to their work with each gang. Calls at night arguably present a greater risk since it is easier to hide and slip away in the darkness. However, their colleague had been shot at in broad daylight.

Think scene surveillance. They would go with their assigned police escort but they themselves also would closely survey open windows, balconies, telephone poles, and mailboxes for possible hiding rival gang members. They would try to account for all persons on the street. However, the neighbors were so frightened that, when a shooting like this one happened, the streets were eerily empty and quiet when the paramedics arrived onsite. After the police had secured the street corner, Mike and Kevin would use a "care and cover" approach with Mike looking for potential rival gang members, and Kevin providing the medical care as quickly as possible. Flashlights would be needed and would be held beside their bodies to avoid creating a silhouetted target. They would park with a clear exit out and they would move as quickly as possible. They had already called the receiving emergency room to alert them to the nature of the call and the potential for violence there as well.

Think old brain stem. Even though these gang members were tough, it was likely that the victim would be thinking in old brain stem due to the sudden shooting, the loss of blood, and/or substance use. Mike and Kevin would announce clearly who they were so the victim did not fear a second gang attack on his person. They would use short words to enhance higher cognitive reasoning but they would also work quickly at the same time to staunch the bleeding.

Think early warning signs. Mike and Kevin knew the warning signs by heart and also knew that gang members, even those medically compromised, can become violent. Under the guise of a quick medical exam, they would search the victim's body for any additional weapons. They would monitor the patient's behavior continuously until they reached the emergency room.

Think theories of violence. Mike and Kevin had actually thought a good deal about the causes of the gang violence that occupied much of their workweek. Certainly, the gangs were operating in a cultural state of anomie, a culture with minimal social cohesiveness and concern for others. They were impressed with the possible sociological explanations: dysfunctional families, poverty, inadequate schooling, discrimination, domestic violence, substance use, and easy access to weapons. Each played a role in this neighborhood disorganization. Other than substance use, the biological theories had less to offer. These young people were not psychotic. Some had attention-deficit hyperactivity disorder, some had abnormal EEG readings, but other persons who had these problems did not become gang members or behave violently. The psychological theories presented a paradox. Both gangs were primarily corporate gangs engaged in selling drugs for profit. The members had to have some business savvy to do this successfully and they were extremely self-disciplined. As such, they demonstrated superior reasonable mastery. Yet at the same time, their interpersonal skills of empathy and nonverbal conflict resolution were next to nil. Over time, the various gang members had appeared motivated by greed, enforcement of their own sense of justice, revenge, hatred, and many of the other base human instincts. All of their sources of motivation appeared to be antisocial.

Think psychological trauma. From past calls, Mike and Kevin know that many of these young gang members had been victims of violence and manifested the hypervigilant, exaggerated startle response, intrusive memories, and avoidant withdrawal symptoms of untreated PTSD. They knew the risk management strategies for approaching trauma victims but the street scenes that they were called to were similar to a war zone, so that many of the risk management strategies were implemented in the ambulance at a later point. Care, cover, and withdrawal to safety were frequently the understandable overriding concern.

Think domestic violence was unlikely to be relevant in the present case. However, *think psychiatric emergencies/substance use/suicide* was highly relevant as regarded substance use. They reviewed the signs of cocaine addiction and the side effects associated with its withdrawal.

Think continuum of youth warning signs. These gang members were poster children for the warning signs of youth violence. These victims had experienced the early warning signs of disruptions in mastery, attachment, and meaning. Most had at least one of the serious warning signs of depression, substance use, and untreated PTSD, and all had the urgent warning signs of conduct disorder and criminal behavior before age fifteen. These gang members likely joined the gangs as family substitutes but their collective interpersonal-skill deficiencies did little to improve the quality of their lives. These gang members had all of the warning signs of youth violence and the aggressive behaviors associated with them. Mike and Kevin knew the youth warning signs, assumed that they would be present in this call for assistance, and took them very seriously.

Mike and Kevin waited three blocks away without lights and sirens, until the police had surveyed the scene and indicated it was safe to drive to the victim. They surveyed the scene a second time and included all of the steps noted above. Mike and Kevin then left their truck to assist the victim. Mike provided cover and Kevin provided care. He instantly recognized the gang insignia and proceeded apace. He applied the tourniquet to the victim's left leg where the main artery had been severed. He also realized the victim was in withdrawal from cocaine. The victim was placed on the stretcher and moved to the medical evacuation unit. Kevin climbed in behind him as the police left. Mike got into the cab and they sped ten blocks to safety. Elapsed time: eleven minutes. Since the victim was now becoming agitated, he was placed in four-point restraints, searched for any additional weapons, and then assessed for any additional medical or psychiatric emergencies. There were no additional emergent situations and they raced to the emergency room that was expecting them.

This was a very potentially deadly situation for the victim as well as the caregivers. By reviewing the guidelines and utilizing the various risk management strategies that were indicated, this run was completed safely. Again for practice, it may be helpful to review the safety guidelines assessment/intervention tool for this case.

Case Example 4: The Impaired Colleague

Susan was the nurse practitioner specialist in emergency care on the hospital medical flight helicopter service. It was Dr. Brown, the pilot, and herself that transported patients with critical care needs. The work was stressful but she loved flying and being of service to others. So much so that she often volunteered for extra flights at the expense of time with her husband and young daughter.

The joy of nursing came to an abrupt end four years ago on the call to the Wellington household. Two children, ages two and five, had been severely burned in an arson fire set by their parents to collect insurance money. As the chopper lifted off from a nearby playground, Dr. Brown and Susan began advanced life support interventions for their victim patients. Each child had third-degree burns over most of its body and it was problematic whether either would survive. Susan thought of her own little girl. The smell of burnt human flesh, the disfigurement of the bodies, added a sense of urgency to the team's work. Susan was assisting with the youngest child, when its face shuddered with intense, almost palpable pain, and the child died.

Susan could not forget that look. She saw the face when she looked at her own daughter each day. The image of the victim's face haunted her working hours and her dreams at night. She was emotionally overwhelmed by the tragedy with no one to speak to, because she did not want to burden the others who were equally upset. Although her mother had been an alcoholic and Susan had vowed as a teenager never to touch alcohol herself, two weeks after the fire, she took a drink to steady her nerves. The psychic pain continued; the drinking increased until four years later she was angry and denigrating of her patients, angry with her colleagues, having strained relations at home, and was continuously depressed. Her anger and professional behavior had become so unpredictable that Dr. Brown was considering removing her from active flight duty for her safety as well as that of everyone else.

What has happened to Susan can and does happen to the very best of those who seek to serve others. A life of service to others, especially steady exposure to potentially violent behavioral emergencies, can be emotionally taxing and physically exhausting. Add to this the stress of normal life, and health-care providers may feel understandably overwhelmed. This is what happened to Susan. She is currently trying to cope with three important issues: untreated PTSD from the death of her young burn-victim, alcohol substance use, and job burnout. Susan is not alone. This triad of problems is often found across the spectrum of all health-care providers. No one in the field is immune from the impact of the life events that we are asked to address.

Untreated PTSD is common among caregivers. Arriving onsite to assist with the impact of violence on the human body is often gruesome and extremely unsettling. People's inhumanity to one another is often unimaginable, unimaginable that is until you are asked to treat its aftermath. Susan was traumatized by the sudden death of her young burn victim, so close in age to her own daughter. Susan was reminded of life's fragility in a special way. No shame in being traumatized; it is a normal human response to sudden, unpredictable, life-threatening events. However, its impact was compounded in the present case because Susan chose to be stoic and suffer alone rather than to burden others. This led to her second problem.

Susan complicated her untreated PTSD by self-medicating her psychological and physiological distress with alcohol. In a few short years, she had become addicted to alcohol, just as her mother was addicted. This substance use led to her irritability and compounded her depression from the young burn victim's death, as depression is also a side effect of alcohol.

Finally, Susan has burnout. This is a particular form of life-stress that may befall those of us who assist others, as noted. Helping people is stressful in that you must assess the need, find a solution, and implement it; and at each stage in the process the person that you seek to help may resist, refuse, or reject your efforts. Over time, people-helping can be extremely draining. This overextension manifests itself in emotional withdrawal from the people that we seek to serve. The withdrawal is followed by an oral denigration of those same persons who have come to us for assistance.

We could ask ourselves how a highly intelligent, highly trained nurse could miss all this turmoil in her own life, how she could overlook the signs of these medical conditions that she had studied in her classes. But in doing so, we would overlook her humanness and her busy life. These issues, untreated PTSD, self-medication with substances, and burnout quietly intrude themselves into our lives like a quiet tide upon the shore. The tide is high before we are fully aware of it. The good news is that each of these issues can be fully remedied.

We turn our attention now to the self-care guidelines: *think self-defense* and *think health and wellness.* Before we implement these guidelines in depth, we need to develop a recovery plan for Susan's three immediate medical issues. We will develop with her a program that proceeds in small manageable steps. There is no preordained timeline for the restoration of her health and well-being and the entire program of both recovery and wellness may take two or three years. In the meantime, each step of the plan will reduce suffering and lay the basis for later optimal health and wellness.

Susan first needs to address her substance use problem with alcohol. Her continued use of alcohol is making her more irritable and depressed, and may in time lead to physical health problems, including memory impairment and a heightened propensity to violence. This alcohol self-medication may also be a way of anesthetizing the intrusive memories associated with the young burn victim's death: but the alcohol is blocking effective recovery from the traumatic incident.

Susan has several choices for recovery and needs to find which is the most comfortable process for her. Going "cold turkey" or stopping on her own is not a good choice because of possible medical complications. She could join Alcoholics Anonymous, she could attend a group for impaired professionals, she could see an addictions specialist, or she could create a combination of any of these approaches. Alcoholism has been a problem in her family and sobriety will be a key factor in restoring her sense of inner peace and contentment.

After a period of sobriety, Susan would then be ready to begin her treatments for the unresolved PTSD. Since this treatment will require her to revisit the memories of the burned child, the initial period of sobriety is crucial since thinking again about what happened at the fire may increase her urge to drink to blot out the psychological pain once again. Susan has a choice of individual or group PTSD treatment. PTSD treatments vary to some degree, but many include a stress reduction program, a psychoeducation discussion of psychological trauma and PTSD, a program on PTSD symptom management, and then an actual review in great detail of the traumatic incident so that it may at last be put to rest.

With these two major issues behind her, Susan may now focus on the third issue: burnout. As noted, burnout is a psychological state that results from the stress of repeatedly responding to people's demands and requests. Teachers, librarians, retail clerks, as well as health care personnel, are all subject to possible burnout. People with burnout are not bad or mean people. They are individuals who are overwhelmed by "people stress" and are psychologically withdrawing as a means of personal self-defense.

The basic treatment for burnout is threefold: develop good stress management skills, change your job description in the near term, and put more fun into your life. Good stress management skills will be outlined in more detail below and can be implemented gradually. They are important in managing burnout because they reduce the physiological arousal level that results from the heightened stress that the individual in burnout has had to deal with for so long. The change in job description, if only for a short time period, is to introduce change in person/people demands, so that the person gets a rest from whatever kinds of people demands that have led to the burnout. For example, Susan might ask to be given some time in working in quality management or on a research project where patient demands for care are less immediate. In time, Susan will be able to resume her med flight-career and enjoy it as she once did. The third leg of this burnout triangle is to have more fun in life. Frequently, it is the more serious, responsible, deadline-meeting person who develops burnout and the person's mind and body eagerly welcome the less purposeful activities of play. The person's mind and body welcome the relief, and human energy is rejuvenated. Susan should not work hard at having fun, as this will defeat the purpose of play.

When Susan has successfully addressed and mastered her three medical concerns, she will be ready for the self-care guidelines to avoid getting into these or similar problems in the future.

Think self-defense. After experiencing the medical issues that Susan has been through, her initial training in self-defense skills may have become tattered at the edges, may have suffered serious decline, or have been forgotten altogether. A similar process may occur in all health-care providers, where there have been no yearly reviews and update of skills. Thus, Susan would want to review her verbal-nonverbal communication skills, her verbal de-escalation skills, her awareness of alternatives to the use of restraints, and the process of actually utilizing restraints as noted in chapter 7. She would also want to review both the theory and practice of her agency's chosen system of nonviolent self-defense. Behavioral emergencies will continue to present themselves in her practice, and she wants to have in place these sound self-defense skills in addition to the safety guidelines with their various risk management protocols.

Finally, Susan needs to *think health and wellness* so that both her practice will flourish and her personal and family life will be meaningful. Susan will want to be mindful of her optimal level of neurological stimulation so that she does not push herself beyond her endurance limits, and she will want to avoid the false cultural assumption that she can have it all, an assumption that pushes many of us beyond our endurance limits. She will want to employ many different right brain activities (such as aerobic exercise, relaxation exercises, and so on) to reduce, and keep reduced, physiological stress. She will want to follow the seven wise lifestyle choices and incorporate the skills of stress-resistant persons as outlined in chapter 8. She will want to find a balance between work, personal, and family time, and adjust her psychological work contract if need be. Finally, when she encounters future behavioral emergencies with the potential for violence or other severe critical incidents, like the death of the burned child, her agency, or she on her own, ought to avail themselves of post-incident crisis intervention procedures, such as the Assaulted Staff Action Program (ASAP; Flannery, 1998). Such interventions prevent, mitigate, or contain the acute psychological distress associated with traumatic incidents. Such interventions, it is hoped, would preclude the development of PTSD, which is what contributed to Susan's distress in the first place. Bolstered by these stress management strategies, Susan's personal and professional lives should be back on track. For practice, begin to design a self-care program for yourself.

This concludes the review of the various safety guidelines and their suggested risk management strategies to preclude or minimize behavioral emergencies from potentially violent persons, and of the self-care strategies for our optimal functioning and well-being. Since we can all get absorbed into our time-scarce lifestyles so quickly, let me close with some thoughts on how to keep things in perspective. Perspective in its own right can make life less stressful and more meaningful, including managing behavioral emergencies. The historians Will and Ariel Durant wrote a ten-volume history of civilization and then a short summary book called *The Lessons of History* (1968) with many of life's most important lessons. It is helpful reading to assist in keeping things in perspective.

Toward that end, let us close with some additional lessons from history, lessons to reflect on as we in care-giving go about our work and our lives:

Life is short
Change is the only constant
Do everything in moderation
Accept what you cannot change
Be concerned for the welfare of others.

Appendix A: *Relaxation Instructions*

I have taught these relaxation exercises to many people. Such exercises are basically right-brain activities. Thus, they lower the whole stress response all at once. In addition, you can use these exercises in public or private without anyone knowing; these exercises are portable and you can take them with you; and best of all there is no cost to purchase them other than your own time in learning to use them. If you used these exercises for as little as ten or fifteen minutes a day, you would feel remarkably better in a short period of time.

The exercises that I will present here are an amalgamation of deep breathing (Benson, 2000), release of muscle tension, and the use of pleasant imagery. I have taught these exercises to thousands of people over the years, and this appears to be the best combination for the greatest number of people. There are several different types of relaxation exercises available and you may want to add in some additional exercises that interest you.

In doing these exercises, you will be safe and in control. If a true emergency arose, your mind and body would immediately rise from the relaxation state, and you would be capable of solving the problem. When some people relax, they feel out of control or have unusual thoughts. Persons who have lived through traumatic situations sometimes feel this way. In their minds, being relaxed means not being vigilant and in control. If you have this response to the exercises, stop doing them and try an aerobic exercise program instead. Aerobic exercise accomplishes similar stress reduction, and you'll feel more in control. If you have lung disease, check with your physician before you begin these exercises.

As I have noted, my relaxation program contains three parts: slow-paced breathing, the cognitive release of muscle tension, and conjuring a pleasant and relaxing image.

Begin with the breathing. Because of the pace of our daily life, we learn to breathe more quickly than we need to. We can slow down our respiration cycle without any serious side effects. The cycle I use in teaching people runs on five-second intervals. Five seconds to inhale a full breath using the whole lung. Five seconds of holding that air. Five seconds of exhaling the air in a slow steady column. Five seconds of sitting quietly without drawing your next breath. Then the twenty-second cycle begins again. Try it now, if you wish. Like any other skill, learning this will take practice. Go at your own pace, but leave time for each of the four intervals, and go more slowly than you normally would. (If you are a smoker, you may have initial difficulty with these exercises.) Five seconds: inhale. Five seconds: hold. Five seconds: exhale. Five seconds: hold. Then begin again.

The second part of these exercises includes the cognitive release of muscle tension in the muscle groups listed below. Our minds are remarkably powerful instruments for coping with stress. If you think of your muscles being released of tension or set free, your brain will in fact release the muscle tension. When you are breathing slowly as outlined above, think of the various muscles in your body to be freed of tension. Think of them being released and they will be. For example, inhale, hold (release the muscle tension in your toes, arches, and heels), exhale, hold. Inhale, hold (release the muscle tension in your ankles, shins, and knees), exhale, hold, and so forth.

Below is a list of the 11 muscle clusters that I teach to others. Do one grouping at a time, and remember to maintain your slower breathing pace.

1. Toes, arches, and heels
2. Ankles, shins, and knees
3. Thighs, buttocks, and anal sphincter
4. Lower back, up the back to the neck and shoulders
5. Abdomen, chest muscles, again up to the neck and shoulders
6. Upper arms, forearms, down to the wrists

7. Each hand, each finger, each fingertip
8. The muscles in each shoulder and all around the base of the neck
9. The whole neck, the tongue, and the jaw
10. The dental cavity, the mouth muscles, and the upper facial cheeks
11. The eye muscles, the forehead, and the top and back of the scalp

Breathe slowly and go through each muscle grouping – one grouping per one respiration cycle. After you have had a chance to practice, you will be able to complete these two parts of the relaxation exercise in about ten to fifteen minutes.

The third component of my approach is the addition of a pleasant and relaxing image. Think of some place you have been that was pleasant or some place that you would like to visit. Make sure the place you choose has no unpleasant memories for you. Do not select that secluded beach where you broke up with your significant other, do not select that breathtaking mountain where you shattered your leg skiing. Make sure your choice is truly pleasant for you.

After you are breathing slowly and rhythmically, and have released all the muscle tension in your body, close your eyes and imagine your special place. Make your image as real as if you were actually there. Whatever you might see or taste or touch or smell if you were really there – be sure to include those things in your image. If your image is unclear or if you have trouble thinking in images, picture yourself floating on a cloud of your favorite color or picture yourself sitting before a curtain blowing in the summer breezes. Imagine your pleasant scene for five minutes. Be sure you continue to breathe slowly, and keep all the muscle tension in your body released. Relax.

With a little practice, these relaxation exercises of breathing slowly, releasing muscle tension, and imagining a relaxing place can be quite effective in reducing stress response. If you have a particularly stressful day, you can do them for ten minutes in the morning, ten minutes at noon, ten minutes at suppertime, and ten minutes before bedtime. These exercises have the added advantage of being flexible in their utilization. If you are anticipating an event that is making you anxious, these exercises can help beforehand. You can also use them when the event is over to return your body to its normal stress-free resting state.

Appendix B: *Guidelines for Aerobic Exercise*

1. See your physician to obtain medical clearance before you begin an aerobic exercise program and always comply with any suggestions or limitations that your physician may give you.
2. Your aerobic exercises should begin with a three-to-five minute warm-up period. Slowly walk or jog or run in place. Bend, stretch, twist, and generally limber up your body. The warm-up period loosens muscles and joints, increases circulation, and helps to prevent injury. Stretch passively your major muscle groups.
3. Now begin your aerobic exercise. Be sure that you have chosen an exercise that is fun for you to do so that you will be motivated to continue. Start in small, gradual, and manageable steps. S*top if you feel faint, pain, or shortness of breath.* A healthful exercise goal to work toward is three twenty-minute periods of such exercise on three different days in any one calendar week.
4. When you have completed your aerobics, finish with a cool-down period. The cool-down period is similar to the warm-up period. Again, for three-to-five minutes, walk about slowly, jog, or run in place slowly. Do some mild stretching for specific muscle groups. The cool-down period allows your body to adjust from your intense exercise to its more normal resting pace.

References and Select Reading

Allen, M. H., (ed.) (2002). *Crisis intervention handbook : Assessment, treatment, and research.* Second Edition. New York: Oxford University Press.

———, Currier, G. W., Hughes, D. H., Docherty, J. P., Carpenter, D., and Ross, R. (2003). Treatment of behavioral emergencies : A summary of the expert consensus guidelines. *Journal of Psychiatric Practice,* 9, 16-38.

American Psychiatric Association (1994). *Diagnostic and statistical manual of mental disorders.* Fourth Edition. Washington, DC: American Psychiatric Press.

Antonovsky, A. (1979). *Health, stress, and coping.* San Francisco: Jossey-Bass.

Archer, J. (ed.) (1994). *Male violence.* New York: Routledge.

Baker, K., and Rubel, Y. R. (eds.) (1980). *Violence and crime in schools.* Thousand Oaks, CA: Sage Publications.

Belloc, N. and Breslow, L. (1973). The relationship of health practices and mortality. *Preventive Medicine,* 2, 67-81.

Benson, H. (2000). *Relaxation response.* New York: Avon Books.

Bondy, B., Buettner, A., and Zill, P. (2006). Genetics of suicide. *Molecular Psychiatry,* 11, 336-51.

Borak, G. (2006). Theories of violence: A critical perspective on violence. In Dekeseredy, W. and Perry, B. *Advanced critical criminology: Theory and application.* Lanham, MD: Lexington Books.

Borum, R., Swartz, M., and Swanson, J. (1996). Assessing and managing violence risks in clinical practice. *Journal of Practical Psychology and Behavioral Health,* July, 205-15.

Bowlby, J. (1982). *Attachment and loss, vol. 1: Attachment.* Second Edition. New York: Basic.

Bouchard, T. J., Jr. (1994). Genes, environment, and personality. *Science, 264,* 1700-1701.

Brenner, H.M. (1973) *Economy and mental health.* Baltimore: Johns Hopkins.

Creeden, K. (2005). Trauma and neurobiology: Considerations for the treatment of sexual behavior problems in children and adolescents. In Longo, R., and Prescott, D. (eds.). *Current perspectives: Working with sexually aggressive youth and youth with sexual behavior problems.* Holyoke, MA: NEARI Press.

Curry, G., and Decker, S. (2003). *Confronting gangs: Crime and community.* Second Edition. Los Angeles: Roxbury Publishing.

Defelm, M. (2006). *Sociological theory and criminological research, vol. 7: Sociology of crime law and deviance.* Oxford: JAI.

DiGrazia, S. (1964). *Of time, work, and leisure.* New York: Anchor.

Drucker, P. (1994). The age of social transformation. *Atlantic Monthly,* 276, 53-80.

Durant, W., and Durant, A. (1968). *The lessons of history.* New York: Simon and Schuster.

Durkheim, É. (1997). *Suicide: A study in sociology.* Trans: Spaulding, J. and Simpson, G. New York: Free Press.

Easton, S., Shostak, M., and Konner, M. (1988). *The Paleolithic prescription: A program of diet and exercise and a design for living.* New York: Harper and Row.

Everly, G. S., and Lating, J. M. (2002). *A clinical guide to the treatment of the human stress response.* New York: Plenum.

Everly, G.S., and Mitchell, J.T. (1999). *Critical incident stress management (CISM): A new era and standard of care in crisis intervention.* Second Edition. Ellicott City, MD: Chevron.

Finklehor, D., and Jones, L. (2006). Why have child maltreatment and child victimization declined? *Journal of Social Issues, 62,* 685-716.

Flannery, R. B. Jr. (1995). *Violence in the workplace.* New York: Crossroad.

——— (1998). *The Assaulted Staff Action Program (ASAP): Coping with the psychological aftermath of violence.* Ellicott, MD: Chevron.

———. (2000). *Violence in America: Coping with drugs, distressed families, inadequate schooling, and acts of hate.* New York: Continuum.

———. (2003). *Becoming Stress-resistant through the project SMART program.* Ellicott, MD: Chevron.

———. (2004a). *Posttraumatic Stress Disorder : The victim's guide to healing and recovery.* Second Edition. Ellicott, MD: Chevron.

———. (2004b). *Preventing youth violence: A guide for parents, teachers, and counselors.* New York: Continuum.

———, Juliano, J., Cronin, S., and Walker, A. P. (2006a). Characteristics of assaultive psychiatric patients: Fifteen-year analysis of the Assaulted Staff Action Program (ASAP). *Psychiatric Quarterly,* 77, 239-49.

———, Walker, A. P., Flannery, G. J. (2006b). Elderly patient assaults: Empirical data from the Assaulted Staff Action Program (ASAP). *International Journal of Emergency Mental Health,* 8, 221-26.

———, White, D. L. , Flannery, G. J., Walker, A. P. (2007). Time of psychiatric patient assaults: Eleven-year analysis of the assaulted staff action program (ASAP). *International Journal of Emergency Mental Health,* in press.

Gelinas, D. J. (1983) The persisting negative effects of incest. *Psychiatry,* 46, 312-32.

Gilligan, J. (1996). *Violence: Our deadly epidemic and its causes.* New York: Putnam.

Guo, G., Roettger, M. E., and Cai, T. (2008). The integration of genetic propensities into social-control models of delinquency and violence among male youths. *American Sociological Review,* 73, 543-68.

Harragan, B. (1977). *Games mother never taught you: Corporate gamesmanship for women.* New York: Rawson.

Herman, J. (1992). *Trauma and recovery: The aftermath of violence from domestic abuse to political terror.* New York: Basic.

Horowitz, L., Kassam-Adams, N., and Bergstein, J. (2001). Mental health aspects of emergency medical services for children: Summary of a consensus conference. *Journal of Pediatric Psychology,* 26, 491-502.

James, T. B. (2003). *Domestic violence: The 12 things that you aren't supposed to know.* Chula Vista, CA: Aventine.

Kempe, C. H., Silverman, F. N, and Steele, B. J. (1962). The battered child syndrome. *Journal of the American Medical Association,* 181, 17-24.

Khantzian, E. J. (1997). The self-medication hypothesis of substance use disorders: A reconsideration of recent applications. *Harvard Review of Psychiatry,* 4, 231-44.

Kindlon, D. (2001). *Too much of a good thing: Raising children of character in an indulgent age.* New York: Hyperion.

Kleepsies, P. M. (ed.) (1998). *Emergencies in mental health practices: Evaluation and management.* New York: Guilford .

Krebs, D. (2003). *When violence erupts: A survival guide for emergency responders.* Sudbury, MA: Jones and Bartlett.

Kübler- Ross, E. (1997). *On death and dying.* New York: Scribner.

Layard, R. (2005). *Happiness: Lessons from a new science.* New York: Penguin.

Levinson, H. (1976). *Psychological man.* Cambridge, MA: Levinson Institute.

Linder, S. (1970). *The harried leisure class.* New York: Columbia University.

Lynch, J. (1977). *The broken heart: The medical consequences of loneliness.* New York: Basic.

———. (2000). *A cry unheard: New insights into the medical consequences of loneliness.* Baltimore: Bancroft Press.

McNally, R. J. (2003). *Remembering trauma.* Cambridge,: Harvard.

Maslow, A. (1962). *Toward a psychology of being.* Princeton: Van Nostrand.

Mann, J. J. (2003). Neurobiology of suicidal behavior. *Nature Reviews. Neuroscience,* 4, 819-28.

Massachusetts Department of Mental Health (2002). *System of nonviolent strategies and de-escalation.* Boston: Massachusetts Department of Mental Health.

Massachusetts Department of Mental Health (2007). *Medication information manual.* Boston: Massachusetts Department of Mental Health.

Mills, L. G. (2003). *Insult to injury: Rethinking our response to intimate abuse.* Princeton: Princeton University.

Mitchell, J. T., and Resnick, H. L. P. (1981). *Emergency response to crisis. A crisis intervention guidebook for emergency services personnel.* Bowie, MD: Robert Brady.

Popenoe, D. (1996). *Life without father: Compelling new evidence that fatherhood and marriage are indispensable for the good of children and society.* New York: Free Press.

Prothrow-Stith, D. (1991). *Deadly consequences.* New York: HarperCollins.

Roberts, A. R. (2000) *Crisis intervention handbook: Assessment, treatment, and research.* Second Edition. New York: Oxford.

Russell, D. E. H. *Rape in marriage.* Second Edition. Bloomington: Indiana, 1990.

Sagan, L. N. (1987). *The health of nations: True causes of sickness and well-being.* New York: Basic.

Schlosser, E. (2001). *Fast food nation: The dark side of the all-American meal.* Boston: Houghton-Mifflin.

Schor, J. B. (1991). *The overworked American: The unexpected decline of leisure.* New York: Basic.

Scitovsky, T. (1976). *The joyless economy.* London: Oxford.

Seigel, D. (1999). *The developing mind: Toward a neurobiology of interpersonal experience.* New York: Guilford

Selye, H. (1956). *The stress of life.* New York: McGraw-Hill.

Stanely, T. J. and Danko, W. D. (1996). *The millionaire next door: The surprising secret of America's wealth.* Atlanta: Longsheet.

Strauss, M. A., and Gelles, R. I. (1992). *Physical violence in American families: Risk factors and adaptations to violence in 8,145 families.* Edited with Smith, Christine. New Brunswick, NJ: Transaction.

Tardiff, K. (1996). *A concise guide to the assessment and management of violent patients.* Second Edition. Washington, DC: American Psychiatric Press.

———. (1998). Unusual diagnoses among violent patients. *The Psychiatric Clinics of North America,* 21, 567-76.

Teicher, M., Andersen, S. L., Polcari, A., Anderson, C., and Navalta, C. (2002). Developmental neurobiology of childhood stress and trauma. *Psychiatric Clinics of North America,* 25, 397-426.

Tracy, P., Wolfgang, M. E., and Figlio, R. M., (1990). *Delinquency careers in two birth cohorts.* New York: Plenum.

Tueth, M. J. (1995). Management of behavioral emergencies. *American Journal of Emergency Medicine,* 13, 334-50.

———, and Zuberi, P. (1999). Life-threatening psychiatric emergencies in the elderly: Overview. *Journal of Geriatric Psychiatry and Neurology,* 12, 60-66.

United States Secret Service and United States Department of Education (2002). *The final report and findings of the safe school initiative.* Washington, DC: Department of Education.

Verney, T. (with Kelly, J.) (1981). *The secret life of the unborn child.* New York: Summit.

Vololch, A., and Snell, L. (1998). *School violence prevention: Strategies to keep schools safe.* Los Angeles: Reason Foundation.

Waldrop, A. E., Hanson, R. F., Resnick, H. S., Kilpatrick, D. G., Naugle, A. E., and Saunders, B. E. (2007). Risk factors for suicidal behavior among a national sample of adolescents: Implications for prevention. *Journal of Traumatic Stress,* 20, 869-79.

Walker, L. (2000). *The battered woman syndrome.* Second Edition. New York: Springer.

Widom, C. S. (1989). The cycle of violence. *Science,* 244, 160-66.

Woititz, J. (1983). *Adult children of alcoholics.* Hollywood, FL: Health Communications.

Wolfgang, M., Figlio, R. M., and S ellin, T. (1972). *Delinquency in a birth cohort.* Chicago: University of Chicago.

Wolman, W. and Colamosca, A. (1997). *The Judas economy: The triumph of capitalism and the betrayal of work.* Reading, MA: Addison-Wesley.

Index

About the Author

Raymond B. Flannery Jr., Ph.D., FAPM, is a licensed clinical psychologist; Associate Clinical Professor of Psychology, Department of Psychiatry, Harvard Medical School; and Adjunct Assistant Professor of Psychiatry, Department of Psychiatry, The University of Massachusetts Medical School.

For over forty-five years, Dr. Flannery has been a counselor and educator of professionals, health care providers, emergency services personnel, businesspersons, and the general public about life stress, psychological trauma, and violence—in the community, in the workplace, and in the home. He is the author of 7 books and is the author of more than 150 peer-reviewed articles in the medical and scientific journals on the topics of stress, violence, and victimization. His work has been translated into several languages.

Dr. Flannery designed and fielded the Assaulted Staff Action Program (ASAP), a voluntary, peer-help, crisis-intervention program for employee victims of violence. For nearly 20 years, he has overseen the development of this program, now including 1,500 ASAP team members on 35 teams in 6 states. ASAP is the most widely researched crisis-intervention program in the world.

In 2005, Dr. Flannery received a lifetime achievement award for excellence in crisis intervention research from the International Critical Incident Stress Foundation.

AMHF

AMERICAN
MENTAL
HEALTH
FOUNDATION
BOOKS

Organized in 1924, the American Mental Health Foundation is dedicated to the welfare of people suffering from emotional problems, with a particular concern for the emotional issues of those with special needs and the elderly.

None of the board members of AMHF receives remuneration. Nevertheless, the costs of promoting research, preparing translations, and disseminating the findings and books of AMHF are high.

All donations and sales of AMHF Books constitute a meaningful contribution to the public good. Please visit our Web site for more information on our work. We thank you for helping improve the lives of our citizens.

American Mental Health Foundation Inc
Post Office Box 3
Riverdale, New York 10471-0003

www.AmericanMentalHealthFoundation.org

www.ingramcontent.com/pod-product-compliance
Lightning Source LLC
LaVergne TN
LVHW070831220926
848486LV00033B/410